Profession and Monopoly

Profession and Monopoly

A Study of Medicine in the United States and Great Britain

JEFFREY LIONEL BERLANT

UNIVERSITY OF CALIFORNIA PRESS
Berkeley · Los Angeles · London

University of California Press
Berkeley and Los Angeles, California

University of California Press, Ltd.
London, England

ISBN 0-520-02734-5
Library of Congress Catalog Card Number: 74-76381
Printed in the United States of America

To My Parents

Acknowledgments

Acknowledgments are always difficult to express in full, so I must let a simple "thank you" suffice. Unmentioned must go the hours of patient listening and attention which I received from so many, and the helpful suggestions and criticisms which they provided.

I would like to thank especially those who have most influenced my general understanding of sociology. Without their teaching, this work would have been of a very different nature. Outstanding among them have been Professors Reinhard Bendix, William Petersen, Joan W. Moore, and R. Stephen Warner. I must also express due gratitude to my fellow graduate students in the Department of Sociology at the University of California, Berkeley, who were also my teachers.

I also thank the members of my doctoral dissertation committee, who saw this manuscript through its growing pains. Professor Guenther Roth, who faithfully served as chairman, and who paid a sharp eye to accurate detail and literacy; Professor Neil J. Smelser, who time and again turned my attention to the cogency of my assumptions; and Professor Arnold I. Kisch, M.D., who helped guide me through the history of the medical profession—all helped elevate the standards of intellectual craftsmanship and scholarship which went into this work.

Thanks are also due to many who helped through discussions of this work and through careful readings of the earlier manuscripts: Dean Sanford Elberg of the Graduate Division at Berkeley; Professors Alvin Gouldner, Norman Scotch, David Levine, and Scott Fuller; and Mark Fishaut, M.D.

Above all, I wish to thank R. Stephen Warner, who provided me with encouragement, friendship, collegial stimulation, and many useful comments. His careful work on Max Weber's sociological studies of religion represents a conver-

gence of thought which has entertained this book throughout.

The editorial staff at the University of California Press,
Grant Barnes and Sheila Levine, have surely also helped
further this book's birth. My association with them has been
cordial and pleasurable.

Appreciation is due as well for the typing contributions
of Ruth Yesian and for Dr. James Bush's technical assistance
at the University of California, San Diego, Department of
Community Medicine, in preparing the manuscript.

And to my wife Jo and my son Jordan I extend a very
grateful apology for the absence this book required at a time
when preciously few hours existed to spend with them.

I have obtained from many a great deal of guidance, help,
and sympathy. The responsibility for the content of the book
that follows, however, I must assume alone; and any errors
herein are mine.

Contents

Introduction

By virtually any criteria, the medical profession in the United States and England must be considered a remarkably successful group. Its wealth, prestige, and influence on public institutions testify to the relative security and permanence of this group as a fixture of modern society. Indeed, its success is so well established that one tends to accept it as common sense that the profession should enjoy such success. Nonetheless, the success of the medical profession as a group is susceptible to sociological inquiry. For the sake of convenience, I shall refer to this inquiry as the problem of the institutionalization of the medical profession.

I shall begin with some methodological considerations and a few disclaimers. I do not intend to explain why doctors practice medicine as they do, but rather why they try to structure their relationships with patients and with each other in certain directions. My task will be to explain how a certain type of social group—a profession—was brought into being and established as an ongoing social enterprise in the face of various social constraints which might have conceivably aborted it. Beyond explaining why certain cultural ideals such as service ("professionalism") have been institutionalized, I intend to explain how the carriers of those ideals have established themselves.

The first chapter will examine one major sociological theory of the professions which purports to explain why certain patterns have been institutionalized among professionals. This is Talcott Parsons' functionalist theory of the medical profession. After stating Parsons' theory, I will carefully compare his claims about what he is doing with what he actually does, criticize the adequacy of his theory for answering the questions he raises, and then criticize the adequacy of his theory for answering the questions of my study.

Having pinpointed the inadequacies of Parsons' theory for

1

my purposes, I will try to apply an alternative explanatory scheme to the problem: Max Weber's theory of monopolization. The second chapter will state his theory of group institutionalization through monopolization and expansion, develop it as necessary to fit the subclass of the professions, and demonstrate its superiority to Parsons' theory as a logically adequate answer to the problem of the institutionalization of the medical profession.

Since logical adequacy is necessary but not sufficient for explanatory adequacy, I will turn also to the historical records of two nations to see how well Weber's theory fits the evidence. I shall study the development of medical ethics, in the third chapter, to investigate the extent to which medical ethics have served as an organizational tool for potentially ordering the conduct of physicians in a monopolistic direction. I am most interested in the status of medical ethics as an instrument of internal domination within the profession, but also as an instrument for dealing with changing external political exigencies of the profession.

In the fourth and fifth chapters, I will examine licensure in the English and American contexts for two general purposes: (1) to understand the manner in which the profession has asserted domination over the medical market (primarily with respect to the limitation of external competition), and (2) to understand the dependence of the structure of the medical profession on political and legal conditions.

In the sixth chapter, I shall analyze a recent proposal for the reform of medical practice in the United States. I will show how reform—indeed, reform to ostensibly demonopolize the profession—can serve as a means for professional organizations to extend domination over medical practitioners, associated health workers, and numerous social institutions, thereby furthering the success of the medical profession as a group.

The substantive chapters will not test Weber's theory as a mere hypothesis, rejecting the theory in total because of inconsistency with certain historical evidence, for I recognize that any theory requires conceptual development to cover reality adequately. Instead, I shall regard Weber's theory as a stimulating start, but one requiring development to retain its illuminating power. I shall use evidence, then, not to reject Weber's perspective but to retain what is useful in the perspective; that is, I will use historical and cross-comparative evidence to advance Weber's theory, not reject it.

The American and British medical professions have not been selected because they "control" certain variables. I have not tried to create a hypothesis to explain why the medical profession has been institutionalized and then to find one social case in which it has been and one in which it has not been in order to test the hypothesis. In both cases, the medical profession has been more or less successfully institutionalized, though in one case, the American profession, institutionalization as a profession occurred relatively late, while in the British case successful institutionalization came very early and then ran into a series of major challenges. In a sense, these national histories are only case studies with which to test the applicability of Weber's concepts. One might argue that other nations might as well have been studied, and in part this argument is acceptable. Study of the profession in other nations in similar depth might very well further develop the theory. The American and British cases, however, are particularly instructive because their medical professions emerged from a common cultural tradition and apparently diverged because of historical and political circumstance. They allow one to see how a common idea—the profession—became institutionalized in different ways in these two nations.

One particularly thorny problem which will repeatedly appear in these chapters is that of the relationship between theoretical assumptions of intention and historical evidence about intention. Weber's theory makes certain assumptions about the wants of men in certain situations and the relationships rationally structured by them to pursue their wants. Applied to the historical record, however, these assumptions do a certain amount of violence to one's desire to make only documentable claims about social reality. One will frequently find it "illuminating" to assume that one knows the intent of social actors in situations in order to understand why they structured relationships in certain ways. One will find that many institutional developments are consistent with evidence that the men involved intended to monopolize. In the chapters to follow, this tension will be resolved in the direction favorable to Weber's theory: I will assume that patterns of monopolization were indeed intended and are monopolistic strategies, not coincidences of history.

For a number of reasons one can skip from pattern to strategy with little alarm. First, I am engaging in sociological analysis and not historiography. Even assuming wrongly that one knows what men intended, one has still gained by better understanding the implications of certain orderings of behavior. Second, and perhaps it is the same point, when one speaks of institutionalization or monopolization, to discuss intentions may be necessary but not sufficient. Even if one *knew* on the basis of overwhelmingly hard evidence that medical leaders intentionally tried to monopolize, one would still have to explain how these intentions were converted into social success. Intent to monopolize, therefore, may be at best only one part and at that the least interesting part of explaining monopolization. It is more important to focus on the tenuous link between intended and accomplished monopolization than on the narrow problem of intention.

Third, one is hard put to say what types of evidence would document intentions from the historically distant past. While one might object to reading motives into certain situations, the alternatives are not particularly attractive either. Deducing intent from conduct is a questionable enterprise, but so is accepting at face value statements about intent made by the men being studied. After all, men may act in a certain way for a wide variety of reasons, and men may prevaricate to protect their interests. We are probably not on much softer ground to assume that we know a priori the intentions of social actors. Of course, I do not even go that far. All I claim to do is to be able to state how a rational hypothetical actor would behave in a certain situation. I am only claiming that I can "understand" the situation as someone in that situation might. This methodological strategy of determining intentions on the basis of knowing the nature of the situation is but an alternative to determining intentions on the basis of observing conduct or obtaining statements of intention. I would feel better, of course, if my historical interpretations were supported consistently by all three types of evidence, but I recognize that I can get along with less than perfect grounding of my theory. While recognizing the persisting uncertain gap between general monopolization strategies and historical patterns merely consistent with monopolistic intent, I propose to try narrowing the remaining gaps between monopolization theory and the historical record.

CHAPTER ONE

Talcott Parsons on the Medical Profession

Because Talcott Parsons is widely esteemed throughout American sociology, his views constitute the major contemporary sociological perspective on the medical profession. Coming from perhaps the most influential living sociologist in the United States and Europe, his conceptual formulation of the profession has tended to dominate serious research in this area. His work on the medical profession is also important inasmuch as it constitutes one of his few pieces of empirical research and provides practical insights into the complex intellectual world of Parsons. By understanding the workings of the medical profession, one might better see the Parsonian view of the workings of society, as though the medical profession were a microcosm of society. These methodological and theoretical aspects of Parsons' work, unquestionably interesting and important for the general sociologist, are nonetheless tangential to the analytical problem of the extent to which Parsons' theory of the medical profession can contribute to one's understanding of the institutionalization of the medical profession.

Parsons' work is relevant in three respects: the adequacy of his proposed answer for the questions which he sets forth, the limits of applicability of his theory, and the adequacy of his theory as a general theory of institutionalization. Certain portions of his argument are acceptable, and the

6

theory cannot be dismissed in its entirety, yet his work requires careful specification and delimitation of its applicability.

Parsons has written three major essays on the medical profession.[1] One, a discussion of professions in general, will not be reviewed, for it is a more general statement of the ideas which Parsons later developed in 1951 in *The Social System* concerning the medical profession. The major body of his thought on the medical profession is contained in his chapter in *The Social System,* but many important insights into his views can also be obtained from his less well known 1965 essay on the medical profession.

Parsons' theory of the medical profession

Essentially, Parsons' theory states that illness creates a situation with certain psychological tensions and that men create norms to reduce these tensions. These norms are oriented toward maximizing the performance of socially useful tasks and, therefore, are functional for maintaining the social system. In the case of the medical profession, the social function is the prevention of "too low a general level of health" and thereby the prevention of dysfunctional incapacitation of members.[2] Illness itself, in this perspective, is defined as those conditions which incapacitate men for meeting their social responsibilities.

Parsons addresses the roles men pattern to deal with the problem of illness. He recognizes that certain men (physicians) are expected to help the ill and, for that matter, that the ill (patients) are expected to cooperate with being helped. The situation of the patient and the physician, however, requires facilitating norms.

What is the situation of the patient? Parsons states that

[1] Talcott Parsons, "The Professions and Social Structure," in *Essays in Sociological Theory* (Rev. Ed., London: The Free Press of Glencoe, Collier-Macmillan, 1954), pp. 34-49; *The Social System* (London: The Free Press of Glencoe, 1951); and "Social Change and Medical Organization in the United States: A Sociological Perspective," in *The Annals of the American Academy of Political and Social Science* 346 (March 1963), pp. 21-33.

[2] Parsons, *Social System*, p. 430.

the patient is helpless and in need of help, yet technically incompetent and emotionally involved. Social institutions recognize that the patient is in a condition requiring help, perhaps through no fault of his own, and entitle the patient to receive help, particularly technically specialized help. The patient is helpless in two major senses: technically incompetent in that he knows less well than a physician how to help himself, and at times physically helpless in that he might not be able to do what needs to be done. Both types of helplessness require the patient to rely on professionals and professional authority, for without technical knowledge a patient cannot rationally evaluate the technical adequacy of physicians. True, a patient may try to judge physicians on the basis of self-assumed knowledge or other criteria, but his doing so only represents the failure of mechanisms for validating the physician's authority. A patient's emotional involvement, from the initial "shock" of illness and then "anxiety about the future," further undermines his capacity for objective judgment. These three elements in the situation of the patient—technical incompetence, physical helplessness, and emotional involvement—combine to make a patient vulnerable, i.e., exploitable and more or less incapable of rational judgment.

The situation of the physician also poses a number of obstacles to helping the ill. First, knowledge may not be adequate for controlling the patient's illness: certain conditions are uncontrollable and every situation contains uncertainty, particularly about the appropriate body of knowledge to apply and the variables which will affect treatment. Second, because of sentiments concerning "inviolability" of the body, the patient may not cooperate. The patient may be excessively modest about nudity and the examination of sexual organs, and he may hesitate over uncomfortable and inconvenient procedures. Third, the physician may be psychologically stressed by confrontation with human illness and death and the knowledge of intimate details of the patient's private life. Despite competence, the physician may at times himself be helpless and emotionally involved, also making objective judgment more difficult.

The solution to the problem which the patient and the physician face is the adoption of problem-solving roles. If the patient is ever to receive help, he must be able to assume a sick role that entitles him to help; the physician must offer help to the patient in an acceptable manner. Parsons therefore focuses for the most part on the institutionalized practices which increase acceptability of services and thereby validate the physician's authority. But he includes other functional considerations as well. These are (1) the application of scientific knowledge to clinical practice, (2) the penetration of the patient's private affairs or "particular nexus," (3) the prevention of countertransference, (4) the protection of the physician's interests, (5) the prevention of exploitation and the building of trust in the patient.

Scientific knowledge is maximized by a universalistic system of recruitment and identification within the profession (that is, according to abstract rules and principles, rather than social origins or the particular individuals involved). In this way, the best minds enter the field and incorporate information from a variety of scientific disciplines to broaden the scientific base of medical practice. At the same time, however, functional specificity (that is, orientation to narrowly specified goals) is invoked to encourage practical specialization so that an individual physician will not spread himself too thin.[3]

Penetration of the patient's private life occurs through a combination of the normative pattern variables of universalism, functional specificity, and affective neutrality. These normative orientations are also supposed to prevent inappropriate penetration into the patient's private life. Fundamentally, the physician gains access to the patient's private life by maximizing trust: emphasizing competence, asking health-related questions, and segregating "the context of professional practice from other contexts." Segregation furthers functional specificity and affective neutrality through a number of mechanisms: privileged communications, not caring for personal family members who are ill, control of

[3] *Ibid.*, pp. 455-456.

sexual arousal, and emotional detachment from patients.[4] These same mechanisms also counteract countertransference which might tempt a physician to enter too deeply into the patient's private life. The physician has many opportunities to "become a personal intimate, a lover, a parent, or a personal enemy," which are all said to subvert objectivity and rational judgment. Functional specificity and affective neutrality are therefore institutional means for dealing with this problem. The psychoanalytic strategy, he states, epitomizes this combination, which can be extended to other areas of medicine as well.[5]

Parsons then turns to the problem of interests. Some practices protect physician interests—for instance, the practice of having a "nurse-chaperone" present during certain phases of the physical examination, such as the gynecological examination. In this particular example, the practice limits countertransference and overinvolvement in the patient's private life but is most useful, from the point of view of the physician's interests, for providing potential witness evidence in case of accusations by the patient about illegitimate violations of the patient's body space and thus for preventing blackmail.[6]

Some practices, Parsons explains, conform to a "collectivity-orientation," an orientation toward serving the interests of the patient, to prevent exploitation of the patient's vulnerability. This aspect of the profession, Parsons states, is what led him to undertake a study of the medical profession. To apply the pattern of the business world to medical practice would be difficult

> where each party to the situation is expected to be oriented to the rational pursuit of his own self-interests, and where there is an approach to the idea of "caveat emptor." In a broad sense it is surely clear that society would not tolerate the privileges which have been vested in the medical profession on such terms. The protection

[4] *Ibid.*, pp. 456-459.
[5] *Ibid.*, pp. 459-462.
[6] *Ibid.*, pp. 458-459.

of the patient against the exploitation of his helplessness, his technical incompetence and his irrationality thus constitutes the most obvious functional significance of the pattern.[7]

The practices that distinguish the profession from business include series of "symbolically significant practices," such as the prohibitions against advertising, bargaining over fees, price competition, prohibitions against refusing patients "on the ground that they are poor 'credit risks,' " and permission to use a "sliding scale" of fees. These practices are said to "for the most part cut off the physician from many immediate opportunities for financial gain which are treated as legitimately open to the businessman." They are intended to maximize "mutual trust" between patient and physician, an essential part of an institutional relationship where the physician is expected to do his best to help the patient and where the patient is expected to reciprocate by doing his best to "cooperate."[8] In summary, the use of a "collectivity—orientation" by the medical profession comes about because of its functional consequences: (1) because society would not permit exploitation of the patient's vulnerability, (2) because certain economic practices symbolically and in actuality prevent exploitation of the patient, and (3) because the performance of the medical task requires that the patient trust his physician, except in those unusual situations where the patient is physically unable to cooperate voluntarily, in which case he becomes an "object" rather than an interacting "subject."

Parsons recognizes the physician's temptation to pursue self-interests and so postulates the existence of social controls to constrain this pursuit. These controls are not formal, however, since formalization would undermine the physician's self-confidence, a situation which might be less functional than occasionally permitting an abuse to slip past. Formalization leads to an emphasis on "technicalities" and "always opens the door for the 'clever lawyer' whether he

[7] *Ibid.,* p. 463.
[8] *Ibid.,* p. 464.

be a District Attorney or merely the 'prosecutor' of the medical society's own Committee on Ethics."[9] So while the physician is expected to conform to a formal body of professional ethics, formal sanctions are avoided. This reason, according to Parsons, explains the medical profession's sparing use of existing official committees on ethics and disciplinary procedures. Instead, the profession uses informal controls of loss of professional standing, withholding of financially desirable connections "such as hospital staff appointments or referrals of patients from other physicians," and loss of "the easy informal 'belongingness' to a group who understand each other as to proper conduct."[10] Parsons sums up the discussion of interest with a very important theoretical qualification: ". . . it is to a physician's self-interest to act contrary to his own self-interest—in an immediate situation, of course, not 'in the long run.' "[11] This paradox, carried out through the informal controls of the profession, is also inherent in the medical relationship itself, since the patient's vulnerability makes a certain measure of trust in the physician necessary for the relationship's existence. In this sense, the physician should be aware that for the patient to seek out or return to a physician is good business as well as a matter of morals.

Critique of Parsons' theory of the medical profession

"Parsons' argument is easily misunderstood. Unfortunately, its purpose is misleadingly stated, and one cannot readily grasp the structure of Parsons' argument if one accepts Parsons' opening statements. He presents it as an attempt to "characterize" the normative structure of the professions. A characterization, however, would be a descriptive argument, and Parsons' theory is more than that. Minimally, it contains an implicit explanatory theory for the institutionalization of the profession's normative structure and in this respect is an explanatory argument. Furthermore, Parsons' characterization of the medical profession is in a num-

[9] *Ibid.*, p. 471.
[10] *Ibid.*, pp. 472-473.
[11] *Ibid.*, p. 473.

ber of respects not an accurate description. Indeed, Parsons'
theory is a philosophical as well as an explanatory argument,
a normative account of what Parsons believes the norms
of the medical profession *should be.*

Parsons is in part responsible for the easy misunder-
standing of the purpose of his essay, precisely because of
his misrepresentation of his task as one of characterization,
and because of his inclusion of information collected from
doctors in the Boston area, seemingly making it appear as
though his essay were empirically based. Consequently, any
criticism which merely attempts to disprove his theory by
providing evidence of failure on the part of the profession
to live up to certain norms misses the mark because it misses
the point of the essay.

Had Parsons been trying to describe the behavior of the
members of the medical profession, he would have used his
series of dichotomous variables, "pattern variables," to show
the presence and interaction of different types of action in
the profession. He would have sought out instances of affectivity in the medical role as well as affective neutrality and
tried to examine the consequences of their coexistence and
interaction. He instead characterizes the entire medical
relationship in terms of one choice among the pairs of pattern
variables: he finds it to be marked by affective neurality,
universalism, functional specificity, achievement-orien-
tation, and collectivity-orientation. Clearly, the object of his
descriptive efforts is the normative structure, not the behavior, of professionals.

Parsons, however, does not stop at a mere description of
the belief structure of the profession; his concept of professionalism is other than the beliefs of the profession. In a
1965 essay, he points to a number of beliefs and norms
espoused by the American medical profession, such as the
importance of an individual fee-for-service system, as "illogical" from the standpoint of professional goals. At times, his
formulation of the essential nature of professionalism is
sufficiently different from that of the existing professions to
constitute a workable criticism of particular policies of the
profession. The logic by which he dissociates the system of

fee-for-service from the profession, for instance, is instructive. In *The Social System,* he at first states: "It may or may not be a good social policy to have the costs of medical care, the means of payment for it and so on settled by the members of the medical profession, as individuals or through organizations."[12] Such matters for him seemingly are irrelevant to the question of the nature of the profession. Later in the same essay, however, he seems to adopt a Weberian belief in the technical superiority of bureaucratic administration, which comes through in a short observation that certain features of professional organization are not logically consistent with a scientific orientation:

> There is a certain formal precision and clarity about the existence of a system of formal rules of behavior and formal mechanisms for their enforcement which seems to bear a certain relationship to scientific precision, so that on the basis of 'cultural congruence' one might expect a system of bureaucratic-legalistic social organization to be particularly congenial to a scientifically trained profession.[13]

He develops this theme further a decade later, at the beginning of the debate over Medicare, in his essay "Social Change and Medical Organization in the United States." The profession's demand to retain an individual fee-for-service system at that time did not appear at all consistent to him with the essence of professionalism. He believed that the individualistic system was necessarily adopted as part and parcel of a decentralized system of health-care delivery, since "the physician was placed as much as any businessman in the position of pricing his own services." Yet this situational contingency, gradually ceasing to exist to the extent that it once did, is not consistent with professionalism and always exists as a latent source of embarrassment for the medical profession:

> In the wisdom of hindsight, we can now see that, from certain points of view, there has been a disturbing paradox concealed in this simple state of affairs....

[12] *Ibid.,* p. 436.
[13] *Ibid.,* pp. 469-470.

Personally, I do not think for a moment that the
critical institutional difference between business and the
profession with respect to the profit motive has been
eliminated. What I do argue is that insistence by the
official spokesmen of 'organized medicine' that the individual fee-for-service mode of organization is the morally
ideal one lays the profession wide open to the charge
that they have abandoned their ancient and honorable
devotion to the welfare of the patient."[14]

He then develops an argument to explain this illogical occur-
rence in terms of the slipping social status of "rank-and-file"
practitioners with respect to the relatively more scientific
academically-based elite within the profession who do not
feel unduly threatened by "bureaucratic interference."[15]

Regardless of what one thinks of Parsons' rather ad hoc
explanation, clearly the direction of his argument is the
dissociation of professionalism from the expressed beliefs of
medicine's offical spokesmen. Similarly, Parsons finds some
of the qualities of the organized group nature of the medical
profession logically inconsistent with his preferred set of
professional virtues and so excludes them from his definition
of professionalism by declaring them to be irrationalities.
Essentially, he takes the position that the social organization
of the profession is irrelevant and that the cultural orientations of only certain elite members of the profession are the
proper field for study. This emphasis on the particular beliefs
of a minority within the profession makes for a peculiar
stance for a sociologist: attention is due to the existing beliefs
of the profession as well as those congruent with Parsons'
theory and to the social organization of the profession as
well as its ideologies.

Parsons' theory, as it becomes apparent, is not a description of the medical profession but a narrower enterprise. His
is a moral analysis which does not undertake a description
of the actual condition of the medical profession and its
relationship to patients but which wishes to draft into being
a set of moral rules that would bring about certain desired

[14] Parsons, "Social Change", p. 29.
[15] *Ibid.*, p. 31.

effects if adhered to. When he cites a norm as part of professionalism, he does not mean that it is adhered to by the members of the profession but that he feels it should be. Other beliefs held by doctors he would dismiss as "illogical." If professionals clearly did not act in accordance with his set of idealized beliefs, he would explain that the system of social controls had been inadequate. In short, the logical structure of Parsons' argument is to discount the world of men who have interests that may at times run counter to a purely conceived medical goal.

Parsons' theory of institutionalization, then, is a moral technician's prescription for norms. He offers that if the medical relationship is to be functional, it should incorporate certain types of norms, which I have discussed. The explanatory part of his theory is contained in the logical relationship between his pattern variables and what he sees as the functional task of medicine. Essentially, the logical requirement for certain norms to maximize certain tasks "explains" the institutionalization of those norms.

A close look at Parsons' theory reveals some inconsistency about which task the medical relationship is supposed to maximize. At times, it seems to be the maximization of an independently and technically defined effective medicine, while at other times it seems to be the maximization of the capacity of social members to perform their social roles. These are, I would suggest, separate tasks, but because they overlap somewhat, Parsons has frequently used them interchangeably. Nonetheless, a proper understanding of Parsons' theory requires an examination first of the nature of the explanatory connection he sees between professional norms and the maximization of effective medicine and then of the connection between these norms and the social role of the medical profession.

The maximization of effective medicine

When Parsons inquires into the problem of which moral commitments are minimally necessary to encourage effective medical services, he answers: the application of scientific competence and the intent to serve the best interests of the patient. He wisely does not claim that these commitments *will* be functional but that they are necessary. One must certainly concede the necessity of competence and good faith for voluntary, rationalized, institutionalized services, but Parsons' argument is then tautological. By definition, providing effective medical services seems impossible without competence and good faith. Technically effective services imply the possession of competence, and the physician must orient himself to the interests of his patients if he is to "serve" them. Any benefits that a patient might obtain from an incompetent, exploitative practitioner can well be dismissed as fortuitous (i.e., dismissed as a happy chance).

From the two major moral requirements of scientific competence and good faith, Parsons deduces or at least selects logically consistent pattern variables. The application of scientific knowledge in objective judgments logically requires affective neutrality, universalism, and functional specificity; to help the patient, knowledge must also be combined with a collectivity-orientation. From these pattern variables, more specific aspects of the medical relationship can be deduced. Because the patient must on occasion provide intimate information, the task is made easier if the physician employs affective neutrality, universalism, and functional specificity. Indeed, the task is made easier because the investigation into the personal life of the patient is presented and justified in terms of its necessity for the intelligent application of scientific competence. It is also made easier if a collectivity-orientation is adopted, so that the patient is less self-protective and guarded, in this case because the patient believes that the physician is performing in good faith. In all such instances, the connection that Parsons draws between these specific pattern variables and certain medical norms and practices is a straightforward, logical deduction from the theoretical assumption of the functional necessity for scientific competence and good faith. On this basis, Parsons has concluded that the medical relationship can be characterized as he suggests.

Certainly, Parsons has the beginnings of a logically consistent analysis of the medical profession in terms of asking which features are functional for the performance of the medical task. There is value to the heuristic application of the question of the functionality of certain beliefs and practices, and this perspective can plausibly relate these phenomena to a larger context. But Parsons has overestimated his powers as a social engineer by prescribing norms, for he repeatedly underestimates the difficulty and complexity of the medical task. Effective medicine requires more than Parsons proposes, and some of the items which he submits for consideration are but tenuously functional. All in all, he simply does not see the larger picture of the problem of medical care.

While Parsons can legitimately claim that certain orientations are necessary in the medical relationship, he should consider the necessity for other orientations which might also characterize the medical relationship. Particularism, for instance, enters into the relationship at times as a functional component of delivering effective care. While the rules of science may be universalistic, they must be properly applied in a particular case; the particularism of which I speak is that of a personal service being performed. Even recruitment, supposedly on the basis of achievement, may require a measure of ascription: in a socially heterogeneous society with polarized ethnic or racial groups, only physicians from certain social groups may be able to treat certain types of patients. White physicians, for instance, may not be able to pass safely into certain Black ghettoes, and such a situation would seem to require recruitment at least in part on an ascriptive basis, if Black physicians were to be trained and made available.

Other orientations are also necessary for inducing the patient to enter the medical relationship and cooperate with the physician. Parsons' attitude is that if the physician emphasizes competence, the formation of objective, scientific judgments, and a concern with the interests of the patient, then the patient will be induced to trust the physician and will cooperate. Trust-inducement devices centering on the scientific components of the relationship, however, may not always build trust. Emotional detachment in particular can be interpreted by the patient as disinterest and excessive impersonality. Too narrow a concept of what are "health-related questions" on the physician's part can lead a patient to believe that the doctor is not really trying to understand the patient's situation. Failure of the physician to become even a little sexually aroused may lead some patients to feel that the physician is not fully human or appreciative of the patient's attributes, thereby driving a block between both.

Parsons fails to mention that trust calls for elements of affectivity, particularism, and functional diffuseness, as well as a collectivity-orientation. Patients may be awed by an atmosphere of highly scientific expertise, but they also want their physician to like them, for that inspires trust that the physician will want to help them. For many patients, then, personal friendship and commitment are believed to be a powerful basis for action in behalf of the patient's interests. Trust in this context tends to call for affectivity, in the sense that the physician actually likes his patient. Liking implies that the physician wants to help the patient for the patient's own sake and will therefore be thorough, careful, and thoughtful. The relationship tends to particularism when the patient wants to be regarded as a special individual and not as an object of scientific manipulation. It also tends to particularism when the patient wants to be seen only by the physician who likes him. It tends toward functional diffuseness by welcoming the extensive and nonconditional involvement that occurs between friends. Trust in the physician and validation of his collectivity-orientation claims, then, often tends to be based on these considerations of personalism. Parsons tries to root the collectivity-orientation in the status honor concept of the profession rather than in sentiments of friendship, and so misses this fundamental strain between scientific competence and trust.

Parsons fails to appreciate the difficulty in the medical relationship of balancing the orientations which he includes among the pattern variables. In some respects, effective medicine calls for the application of science with its distinctive set of pattern variables; in others, it calls for the application of trust-inducing methods that are sometimes compatible with the pattern variables of science and are sometimes not. Parsons seriously underestimates the problem of the physician's emotional reaction to the medical setting when he accepts the belief that affective neutrality always furthers the patient's interests and stabilizes the relationship. The degree of emotional involvement that would most help the patient depends on a wide range of factors, including the patient's disease, his psychic set, the family's reaction, and the reactions of other health personnel. At times, affective neutrality may be most effective, but its value is situation-specific. As much can be said for the other pattern variables.

The point is that considerations to which Parsons does not pay attention also determine the delivery of care. Their significance requires some analysis. The existence of pressures for impersonality in the medical relationship does not reduce pressures for personalism. Each applied appropriately contributes to effective medicine. Theoretically, therefore, there is a certain range of complementarity of both sets of pattern variables in the medical relationship. The problem with Parsons' attempt to generalize from the pattern variables which are minimally necessary for certain specific aspects of the medical relationship to a characterization of the entire relationship is not just a logical error; unthinking application of these orientations throughout the relationship could be quite dysfunctional. Parsons' unqualified philosophical advice can be dangerous for the patient.

Even the appropriate application of these orientations may at times be dysfunctional. An orientation of affective neutrality, for instance, does not call on the physician to stop having emotional reactions; it demands that he behave *as though* he were emotionally univolved. The particular mechanism of compliance with this demand and the personal cost of compliance for physician and patient alike, however, are not clear. One mechanism of compliance might be "hardening" toward the situation of the patient, which constitutes an actual change in emotional response. This mechanism can be dysfunctional by allowing the physician to be more or less indifferent to the feelings and interests of the patient. Another mechanism might retain empathy with the patient's plight, in which certain considerations of affectivity enter into judgment-making.

One of Parsons' few concrete examples can help to clarify the issue:

> An eminent surgeon, for instance, was acutely aware of the emotional reaction provoked in himself by seeing a patient through a long and difficult convalescence from a severe and dangerous operation—one case was a nine-year-old boy. He said he would distrust his own judgment if he had to decide to operate a second time on such a case: He was afraid he would lean over backwards to spare the patient the suffering he knew would be involved, even in a case where he also knew the operation would probably be best for the patient in the long run.[16]

Parsons implies that the professional's moral commitment is to the long run course, that is, to do everything possible to bring about a cure or some stable level of compensation for the disease process. It is as though Parsons were saying, "Of course, the operation should be done; the boy should be saved or helped if at all possible." But the possibility that the operation should *not* be done remains. One possible outcome of the operation may be that the boy will go on to recovery, but another possible course is severe surgical trauma with suffering, pain, and anxious depression culminated by death. The question can be legitimately raised about the basis on which such suffering would be justified. If the physician knew that the boy were going to die, he might well have rejected surgery. As it is, the physician must form a statistical judgment about the probability of recovery and weigh it against the cost of suffering. Even a sure recovery might have to be bought at such a high cost of suffering that the operation might be thought not worthwhile. Perhaps the physician whom Parsons describes should not have mis-

[16] Parsons, *Social System*, p. 458.

trusted his own judgment. Not doing the operation might be considered kinder. Such humanistic considerations are often more important to the patient and his family than purely technical ones of "doing all that can be done." In this regard, then, Parsons' physician who would have leaned over backward to avoid surgery might well be considered superior to the one who did not consider the patient's suffering. The charge that he might make the "wrong" decision only begs the question of what the "right" one would be. Obviously, the assumption of such responsibility for another person's fate can be distressing for the physician. The personal cost for the physician of adopting this particular mechanism of "affective neutrality" may be very high, and the possibility should be considered that it can be dysfunctional for the medical relationship in the long run, perhaps by altering the physician's psychological set or by making practice intolerable for him. One can only wonder how Parsons' tormented physician would have felt if the boy had died following surgery and what long-term effect such incidents would have had on his practice.

Parsons' discussion of the functional requirements of the medical relationship for the maximization of effective medicine overlooks the complexities of inducing patients into the relationship, as well as the multiple difficulties of determining what constitutes effective medicine. Obviously, the application of scientific thought in medicine stands in some conflict with the practical delivery of care on an interpersonal level, and it is not sufficient for the physician to be merely "scientific." He must come to terms at all times with the particular emotional, personal, and philosophical biases of his patients, or he will risk the breakdown of his relationship with the patient. Even so, the persistence of the medical relationship is not an end in itself, and the question of the role of the medical relationship becomes a serious concern.

The social role of medical services

The basic functionalist position in Parsons' argument is that the medical relationship is related to the functional requirement of the maintenance of the social system. Such maintenance requires the capacity to fulfill roles. So, a role relationship is created to minimize incapacity: the medical relationship formed by the interacting roles of physician and patient. If the role relationship is to work and system maintenance be furthered, certain orientations are necessary, because effective medicine requires certain elements. "Effective" is defined here as any therapy that helps maintain occupancy and performance of system roles. Such a definition, however, employs a social utilitarianism that conflicts with the usually understood individual utilitarianism of the medical profession. The distinction is between efforts to maximize the number who receive benefits and efforts to bring the most benefits to a specific individual. While individual and social utilitarianism may at times coincide, they conflict at several points.

The argument that the maintenance of the social system requires the capacity to fulfill roles, for instance, may well be consistent with social but not individual utilitarianism. People medically classified as "sick" may well perform their roles. If the concept of illness is extended to include psychological phenomena such as neurosis, one might even argue that many roles require a certain amount of neurosis for occupancy and performance, the physician's role possibly being an excellent example. An argument might be made, indeed, that the maintenance of the social system requires a certain amount of incapacitation of the individual's psychic and biological systems. Society runs at a psychological and physical benefit for some, but only at the expense of others. Moreover, social systems exhibit a variable capacity to accommodate to the fact that members become ill and die; the dissociation of the maintenance of the social system from the survival of individual members is in fact part of the process of institutionalization of certain action patterns. The concepts of impersonal office, succession, and authority on the basis of rules, for example, are very important cases of this dissociation. A role relationship created to maintain the capacity of individuals to occupy roles signifies a functional alternative to complete dissociation of roles from particular occupants, and hence represents a stopgap measure. It represents a response to an imperfect institutionalization of the social system. Seemingly, the health of individual members *can* be defined independently of their functional capacity for the system, and at times individuals may make a claim against the system, so to speak, for their own health. Perhaps this claim results in the nonoccupancy of certain roles or the lowering of social productivity; there are, in any case, some areas in which individual health needs do not coincide with the maintenance of the social system.

The argument that the role relationship, medicine, is created to minimize incapacity is misleading. That medical treatment may indeed minimize incapacity and return individuals to their roles is but one consideration. In general, most rationally controlled incapacity is prevented by public health measures, ranging from mechanical considerations such as sanitation to quasi-medical activities such as vaccinations. Reduction in incapacity is probably due to improved conditions of living, in particular better nutrition. René Dubos, an authority in the field of microbiology and public health, attributes very little credit to physicians for the general improvement of health in certain Western nations.[17] These considerations suggest that the maintenance of role capacity is possibly a minor function of the medical relationship, and that it is the individual rather than social utility of medicine that has been institutionally and ideologically important. If definitions of health are considered, for instance, it would seem that a "return to normal life" is only one definition of health currently used. Often, the idea of getting the patient out of his "normal" life and into a less destructive way of life is used. But even when the idea of a return to normal life is employed, it may be justified in terms of the patient's wants or the best available alternatives.

The point is that the medical profession rarely defines its professional goal as the maintenance of the social system; rather, it consistently emphasizes the importance of the health of the patient as an end in itself. Its ideological formulation is so strongly individually utilitarian, in fact, that the bulk of the medical profession has traditionally been

[17] René Dubois, *Mirage of Health* (Garden City, New York: Anchor Books, Doubleday & Company, 1961), pp. 139-140.

opposed to or indifferent to a wide range of public health activities. Parsons, put into perspective, seems to have adopted an idiosyncratic view of medicine with more or less totalistic overtones. His attempt to define health in terms of the individual's functional value for society is, in fact, an ancient alternative to the Hippocratic tradition that places the patient's health above sociopolitical demand, and represents an ideological challenge to the dominant tradition of Western medicine.[18]

The individual utilitarian ethic in medicine permeates the conventionally stated social role of the medical relationship. Parsons has dismissed the central role of the alleviation of suffering in medicine by arbitrarily claiming that "it still seems correct to say that compassion for suffering is less prominent in our attitude complex than is concern about unnecessary incapacity."[19] Incapacity, to him, is more prominent because it represents the waste of a potential social resource and because, through no fault of the individual, it limits upward mobility on the basis of achievement.[20] But the patient whose incapacity is corrected or compensated for may not also have his pain alleviated. A large class of patients represent therapeutic challenges in that they can receive no available effective treatment or can be given only palliative care. Especially with the growth of a proportionately older population with difficult chronic degenerative diseases, and of the capacity of modern medicine to keep alive certain people with handicaps who might otherwise have died, physicians have had to deal more with a population of patients who cannot be expected to return to their normal roles.

Such patients have not always been the objects of medical attention. During the Middle Ages, for instance, treating incurable or hopeless patients was considered unethical and exploitative. Only since the Enlightenment has palliative treatment been regarded as at least as important as curing. Today the most important problems of medical organization

[18] Lain Entralgo, *Doctor and Patient*, trans. from Spanish by Frances Partridge (London: World University Library, Weidenfeld and Nicholson, 1969), pp. 40-41.

[19] Parsons, *Social System*, p. 23.

[20] *Ibid.*

seem to center around care for those who promise little chance of being cured. Palliative treatment may not be of more concern than relieving incapacity, but it is at least as important unless one adopts a strict social utilitarianism. Another relevant observation is that the medical relationship was created and maintained long before it was able to correct role incapacitation to any appreciable degree. When one examines the types of people treated in ancient Greece, for example, one sees that medicine was either bought as a personal commodity by wealthier, privileged strata or as a means for maintaining the functional value of slaves. In the latter case, treatment was administered by a special lower class of medical personnel, a prototypical ancient physician's assistant.[21] The medical relationship, then, appears to have commonly incorporated both individual and social utilitarian aspects, with one aspect predominating over the other in different contexts. It has served both as the expression of a more or less somatized salvation wish and as a means of maintaining the productive utility of subordinated people. Parsons does not seem to appreciate the tension between these two orientations within medicine.

Essentially, Parsons' social utilitarian view of the value of the first four orientations—affective neutrality, functional specificity, achievement, and universalism—runs aground on the individual utilitarian requirements of medicine; and the fifth orientation—collectivity-orientation—similarly cannot be readily accepted on these terms. It is interesting, then, that Parsons does not discuss it in the social utilitarian terms of the rest of his argument.

Parsons' formal presentation of the concept of a collectivity-orientation is, certainly, consistent with social utilitarianism. A collectivity-orientation is not synonymous with altruism; sacrifice on the part of the physician (or other actor) is not demanded. Instead, Parsons defines it as an obligation to pursue the common interests of the collectivity in contrast to "private interests."[22]

[21] Entralgo, op. cit., pp. 30-38.
[22] Parsons, Social System, p. 60.

We would only speak of a role as collectivity-oriented if the pursuit of certain private interests which were relevant possibilities in the given type of situation was subordinated to the collective interest. Thus the public official has an interest in his own financial well-being, which for example he may take into account in deciding between jobs, but he is expected not to take this into consideration in his specific decisions respecting public policy where the two potentially conflict.[23]

Parsons' social utilitarian argument does not address the question of motivational entrance into the role relationship, particularly motivation on the part of the patient. Understandably, physicians can help strengthen the patient's inner psychological resources, correct certain physical problems and return the patient to role-fulfilling capacity. But the relationship between the patient's role compliance and the patient's interests is unclear. Parsons implies that physicians act as moral agents who use all means at their disposal when necessary to persuade the patient to get by with a lower level of gratification or to seek alternative gratifications. Parsons is particularly interested in patients who do not want to get well and in those features of illness that psychoanalysts have termed "secondary gain." Hence, he has constructed a theory, which he describes as characteristic of all medical practice, on the basis of this special type of problem in which the patient's wants are deliberately discounted. By so doing, he avoids building a theory which might explain institutionalization in terms of the interests of the parties involved. In the process, however, he misses several considerations related to the interests of patients and physician alike. Probably the vast majority of patients seek out help not because *society* does not want them to be ill but because *they* do not want to be ill. As far as these patients are concerned, the physician is obligated to meet their interests, not those of the system. The physician may then face a set of potentially conflicting obligations imposed by patients and

[23] *Ibid.*, p. 61.

representatives of the system. Perhaps a hypothetical totalitarian society would consistently demand that physicians ignore their patient's interests in favor of the system, but only in this extreme case does the model seem to be adequate as an explanation.

Out of keeping with a strictly functionalist explanation, Parsons frames most of his actual analysis of medical norms and practices in terms of the satisfaction of the patient's interests, not of society's functional requirements. It is an analysis set in terms of interests and not obligations, particularly from the point of view of the patient: patients enter into and submit to their physician's advice because they want help as defined in terms of their own interests and because they come to trust their physician, not because they are admonished. Patients might be urged to trust their physician, and some physicians even expect trust from patients, but in general no *patient* is morally obliged to trust: trust as a concept is based on the physician's one-sided moral obligation to protect and meet the interests of the one who trusts. If moral obligation were the crucial element, physicians would attempt to curry a sense of moral *duty* on the part of patients, not *trust*.

The social role of medical services as a theory of institutionalization

Parsons' working theory of the medical relationship, then, to a large extent emphasizes the interest component of the patient as a crucial factor. The task of medicine is usually constructed to meet the interests of the patient. In this regard Parsons is aware that the patient is in a vulnerable position on a number of counts. Many of the institutional practices Parsons cites possess a significant potential for coping with patient vulnerability in a number of senses. Patients are medically incompetent, so scientific knowledge is applied to counter their ignorance. The situation of illness is emotion-laden, so affective neutrality is called upon to dampen it. Patients are vulnerable in that they cannot evaluate the need for or the quality of the services provided them, so physicians should adopt a collectivity-orientation. In short, because the patient is vulnerable, the physician should protect the patient. The patient may then remain ignorant and emotional as long as he trusts the physician.

Despite Parsons' manifest social utilitarianism, his argument amounts to an individual utilitarian theory of the institutionalization of the medical profession. In part, this paradox is due to the strongly individual utilitarian ideologies of the medical profession in Western nations. But a more important consideration is that Parsons tends to assume a harmony of interests between individuals and society at large and disregards the distinction between social and individual utilitarianism. He might like to say that the moral demands of society also benefit the interests of patients, but such is not always the case. All that he can say is that the protection of the interests of patients as individuals requires certain orientations, norms, and practices. As a theory of institutionalization, Parsons' actual argument is constructed around the explanatory power of the necessity for the physician as a professional to protect the patient's interests if the patient's interests are to be protected at all. This insight is an important one and, within Parsons' approach, valid as a statement of necessity. As a theory of institutionalization, however, it leaves a number of considerations untouched and a number of questions unasked.

While it is true that effective medicine requires the medical profession to protect the interests of patients because of their vulnerability, there are additional considerations related to the problem of interests, protection, and the institutionalization of certain practices. First, even though the good will of physicians cannot be done without, it cannot always be depended on to exist. There always is a certain degree of imperfect internalization of morals. Those who might come under a code of standards respond personally to the code in a variety of ways. Some may outrightly reject and denounce the code. Others may acknowledge its sanctity and moral correctness, only to give it lip service and ignore it in practice. Others may by and large ignore it most of the time but occasionally perform token gestures. Some may deeply internalize the code and try to adhere to it, but only passively, following the letter of the code in whatever situation they find themselves in. Still others may internalize the code to the extent of being actively compelled to change the situation to further the spirit of the code. There is, in short, a distribution of internalization of morals. Parsons is implicitly aware of this problem and tries to argue that such imperfection is constrained by the informal pressures of the medical profession. He does not, however, provide any reason why the medical profession should enforce a more deeply internalized moral sense than the bulk of its members already possesses. He is confident about the degree to which the profession as a collectivity is willing to protect the interests of patients, but he provides no basis for this confidence.

Essentially, the argument that the profession will make up for the moral deficits of its members is a subclass of the assumption that the professional has truly internalized the norms of professionalism. Despite being framed in terms of norms, the argument is still an attempt to explain the behavior of physicians in terms of the interests of patients. While one may grant that effective medicine requires physicians to intentionally act in behalf of patient interests, it also requires patient self-protection because of the existence of imperfect internalization on the part of the profession and its members. Consistent with such a strategy is the reduction of the knowledge gap between physician and patient to help the patient take a more rational part in his own treatment and the course, and introduction of means for defusing the patient's emotional reaction. It requires the patient to make some sort of effort at protecting his interests, pehaps by getting independent medical opinions or by adopting some other form of comparative shopping. Such a strategy is not merely an alternative structural means for attaining the same end for the patient, but a compensatory mechanism for the increased vulnerability that professionalism imposes on the patient. The introduction of scientific competence which helps increase the potential for more effective care also makes the patient even more incompetent to judge the care he receives. Moreover, those norms and practices that induce trust in the patient may well be deceptive in the presence of imperfect internalization.

The claim that the physician will serve the patient's interests is a powerful inducement for the patient to enter the medical relationship, and in this respect the collectivity-orientation is an important trust-inducement mechanism. There is, however, the problem of misplaced trust. The medical profession demands from current and potential patients a tacit belief in the physician's statements about the reality of the patient's situation. Therefore, professional advice is allegedly "disinterested." Yet a used-car salesman might testify to a customer that he wants to help the customer make a good choice and find a car to serve him well. In both cases the patient and the customer may have the experience of being disappointed with the results of their "purchase." But the unique ideological position of the medical profession is to place itself above the criticisms of those they ostensibly serve by declaring such criticisms illegitimate. The customer may be said to have been "taken," but the patient is said to have not understood. I am not arguing that the collectivity-orientation is a deliberate attempt to mislead the public by false promises, or that physicians are not capable of living up to their ideals. All I mean is that the vulnerability of the patient is heightened when he accepts the profession's claims. While at some point the patient must decide to trust the professional if he is to get professional help, there is certainly no guarantee that this will not be misplaced trust. For patients to construct institutions to help protect their own interests would appear to be rational from their interest position. A patient might be wise to be suspicious of physicians and to apply pressure wherever he can to protect himself. Cooperation with the physician might be deferred until more rational understanding of the situation was attained by the patient, perhaps by obtaining multiple opinions, and until alternative resources had been investigated. If the patient is desperate enough, he might cooperate even if trust and understanding were minimal. The request by the physician for patient trust, however, is in certain respects a request for the patient to remain ignorant and helpless, i.e., dependent. It increases the physician's potential control over the patient as it increases the potential for exploitation.

A second consideration, along with the necessity for patient self-protection of interests, is the necessity for the profession to protect its own collective interests. Minimally, this necessity is due to the material requirements for group existence. Parsons is aware of the concept that professionals pursue their own interests, but he introduces it only as a qualifying phrase:

> It may rightly be said that just as every actor must both have immediate gratifications and accept discipline, so must every role both provide for pursuit of private interests and ensure the interest of the collectivity. This circumstance is not a paradox, because, defined as a matter of orientation-primacy in role-expectations these alternatives apply to specifically relevant selection-contexts, not necessarily to every specific act within the role.[24]

While certainly a professional's personal interests will at many places enter the relationship, it is misleadingly simple as stated. What is interesting is the concept that the collective interests of the profession can play an important part in structuring the medical relationship. The physician may face a choice regarding whose interests should be gratified other than the one between self-orientation and collectivity-orientation. There can be a choice between his own personal interests and the interests of the group (the profession) to which he belongs. He can choose to attempt to gratify his interests as defined in a context of individualistic action or as defined by the particular type of organization that those like him select for the collective pursuit of their somewhat similar interests. The persistence of a profession as a group rather than as an aggregate of professionals, then, requires an orientation toward self-gratification that is group-mediated rather than individual-mediated. In this instance as in

[24] *Ibid.*, pp. 60-61.

regard to professionalism, the institutionalization of the profession, i.e., its acquisition of permanence, is more than the internalization of attitudes by members or the satisfaction of individual ends. Parsons tends to equate these issues and so confuses his levels of analysis.

A third additional consideration is that the morally obligated protection of the patient's medical interests does not include his economic or social interests. Parsons argues that a number of practices, such as privileged communication and the sliding scale, are functional in that they remove social or economic barriers to the patient's entering the medical relationship. These practices, then, are not meant to be used to be kind to the patient but instead to bring him under the physician's control even if he is poor. Parsons appreciates the complementarity of exchanging medical services for payment in money but apparently overlooks the exclusion of economic matters from his study of the relationship by his definition of the collectivity-orientation in terms of the effectiveness of providing medical services. The relationship is characterized by a collectivity-orientation to the extent that action is oriented toward service and not profit. Service, however, can be provided at either high or low cost to the patient and still be considered consistent with a collectivity-orientation. The problem is that patients have economic as well as strictly medical interests, and when one discusses the mutual pursuit of interests, the existence of areas of interest conflict must be considered. Strictly speaking, since the minimal cost to the patient would be free services, any charge made by a professional is at the expense of the patient's economic interests. In this sense, at least within a fee-for-service system, the profession cannot adopt a truly comprehensive collectivity-orientation that encompasses all of the patient's interests, for the profession must also protect its own collective interests. The existence of economic conflict means that in practice the profession may tend to maximize its economic gains while patients may tend to minimize their expenditures.

Some pertinent insights are provided by the analytical distinction between a collectivity-orientation and economic rationality. The "sliding scale" (fee discrimination) and acceptance of poor credit risks constitute a collectivity-orientation with respect to effective medical services but are not always economically advantageous to the patient, because the population from which these patients are drawn presumably would not have otherwise obtained medical services. In the extreme, the poor patient, of course, pays more with a sliding scale than he would have had he received no medical care at all. In terms of the patient's overall economic condition, the patient is poor when he receives care under such conditions. That he might also be healthier is economically irrelevant, at least in the short run. Such logic can be applied to the physician's circumstance as well. If the physician loses income by foregoing treatment of wealthier patients, then the sliding scale represents an altruistic act. If he is not a busy doctor, the sliding scale implies an income increment of some sort without loss of prestige, an increment that might be foregone if the physician were to wait to get his price. So under certain conditions the sliding scale need not be altruistic in an economic sense, and the prestigious benefits of compliance with Christian values of beneficence to the poor can be claimed as well. From the patient's point of view, only the patient who would have purchased services even without a sliding-scale reduction benefits from the sliding scale. In such an instance, the sliding scale has little to do with what a patient can "afford," since he could afford care even at a higher price. For such patients the sliding scale is an economically altruistic device only in the restricted sense that the physician charges less than he might force from his market position. Such altruism, however, falls outside of a collectivity-orientation, since the patient would have entered the medical relationship and received services even without discount. The point is that while Parsons is correct that a collectivity-orientation is not altruism, issues of economic rationality are still important in the structuring of the medical relationship.

The considerations of imperfect internalization, group maintenance, and the independence of economic rationality from the collectivity-orientation suggest a number of important qualifications of Parsons' argument. First, the argument that the profession must assume a moral obligation to protect the interests of patients if their interests are to be protected is probably true. But as has been seen, the profession uses devices that increase the vulnerability of patients and expose them further to the threat of imperfect internalization of morals. One would expect to see the development of institutions and practices on the part of patients to protect themselves, particularly on an organized basis. One would also expect to see physicians help reduce the vulnerability of patients by mechanisms that make trust less necessary in the medical relationship. Very little in these last two respects appear to have occurred in Western nations. Indeed, the systematic disregard for the necessity for patient self-protection constitutes an elitist bias in Parsons' theory. Both the medical profession and Parsons are overly inclined to accept the honorability and reliability of professionals a priori.

Second, even if the fundamental honorability of professionals is assumed, there still remain considerations of group interests. If physicians indeed give disinterested advice, as professionalism would call on them to do, the problem of meeting their own interests is heightened. If they take seriously such norms as the sliding scale and the acceptance of poor credit risks, they might operate at a consistent loss and go out of business. One way of dealing with such strains is to permit practice only in situations that protect the interests of the profession while the code is being applied. The sliding scale, for instance, has been circumscribed by the practice of giving physicians the right to accept only patients they want, except in emergencies. The effect has been to maintain a sliding scale but to distribute care to the wealthier sector of the population. Also, the sliding scale has not been one of the commonly employed or preferred economic devices of the medical profession, particularly in the United States. While the call for a sliding scale has been issued since medieval times, the official profession has typically favored a traditional scale of uniform fees both in

England and the United States.[25] Medical ethical codes in America prior to the past fifteen years have omitted the concept of the sliding scale. The earliest American codes called for uniform fees, and later codes have omitted mention of fee practices altogether. The current code might be construed as favoring a sliding scale, but it too presupposes a fundamental infrastructure of uniform or "fair" fees: it asks that fees be commensurate with the services provided and with the ability of the patient to pay. Similarly, no prohibition against the rejection of poor credit risks has ever been published in any medical code of ethics, either in England or the United States.

Third, some of the practices that Parsons included among his list of collectivity-orientation appear to have less to do with this orientation than with economic rationality. His argument, for instance, that the prohibitions against advertising, bargaining, and price competition are examples of collectivity-orientation is not very convincing. On one level these practices are intended to symbolically differentiate overtly professionals from profit-seeking businessmen; they are supposed to deny the economic rationality of the practitioner. But this symbolism is dependent on the conventional usage of these practices by practitioners otherwise believed competent and trustworthy; their reliability is not established but rather identified by these practices. On a different level are arguments that these practices directly contribute to the protection of the patient's economic interests, in a sense a superfluous argument, since a collectivity-orientation does not preclude economic rationality. Physicians can at times both provide effective medical services and maximize profit by careful segregation of these two activities into different parts of the medical relationship. Carr-Saunders and Wilson, for instance, suggest that advertising might lead patients away from competent practitioners.[26] While this argument might hold in a prelicensure age, licensing has provided a more guarantied form for determining which

[25] A. M. Carr-Saunders, and P. A. Wilson, *The Professions* (Oxford: The Clarendon Press, 1933), pp. 451-542.
[26] *Ibid.*, p. 437.

practitioners are competent. The persistence of opposition to advertising seems to have more to do with the discouragement of economic competition among practitioners. The practices Parsons cites do not even protect the patient's economic interests. Advertising, bargaining, and price competition are all methods for reducing prices and are therefore economically rational for the patient. Prohibiting these practices exposes the patient to the risk of paying high rather than low fees and raises the question of economic exploitation. The use of advertising might not be the clearest example, because it raises operating costs and can be used to make qualitative claims; but insofar as it is a method of price competition, it can be economically rational for the patient.

On many counts, then, the institutional devices of the medical profession can be seen to greatly increase the vulnerability of the patient in the name of reducing it. The unknown factor is the degree of moral internalization. Parsons, too, is sensitive to this problem, though perhaps in a more oblique fashion. His discussion of informal group pressures within the profession focuses on the control of deviance by physicians. The use of informal group pressures, however, raises more questions than it answers. While such pressures might be used to protect the interests of the patient, they might also be used to maximize adherence to a set of standards which is only selectively enforced. The fact that such pressures might be used to protect the patient does not mean that they will be. They might well be used to enforce verbal acknowledgment, i.e., to institutionalize the cultural code without regulating more than token compliant behavior. And even if group pressures were used to maintain a collectivity-orientation with respect to the medical interests of the patient, the question of the relationship of group pressures to the pursuit of economic interests remains unanswered: to what extent are group pressures oriented to the maximization of economic gain?

Nothing about the economic incentives of a fee-for-service system would induce the profession to follow the collectivity-orientation. Obviously, a strong group economic incentive exists to perform services, for these further the economic

interests of members; yet services are not necessarily performed in behalf of the patient's interests. The tying of
payments to the performance of "services," in fact, increases
the vulnerability of the patient by creating an economic
incentive to perform medically unjustifiable or marginally
justifiable services in certain instances. The only obvious
benefit that an economic incentive of this sort can be said
to bring about is to increase the quantity of services provided,
or, as the medical profession usually expresses the sentiment,
to get the physician to "work harder." It cannot easily act
as an incentive for higher quality work; in fact, it acts as
an incentive against it, not only in the gross sense of con-
sciously violating the sentiment outwardly expressed in the
statement of a collectivity-orientation, but also in a more
subtle way. Since a higher price can be placed on certain
services, the physician can obtain higher profits by preferen-
tially choosing them. More expensive services are usually
defended as more difficult to perform, more complex, and
in general requiring more responsibility. A constant economic
pressure exists, then, to push practice to the limits of competence and perhaps in some cases to exceed them. Also, many
physicians are reluctant to perform time-consuming simple
services, which are often intellectually unrewarding as well
as relatively less financially rewarding, and the economic
incentive structure supports this reluctance. I see, therefore,
no clear reason why economic incentives should lead the
individual practitioner to internalize the collectivity-orientation and "live up to it." Nor is seeing that colleagues
actually help patients necessarily economically advantageous for practitioners as a collectivity. Only considerations
of salability of services are relevant, and precisely this relationship between salability and utility is at question.

Creating "good will" in the medical marketplace is problematic, for it can be based on illusion as well as actual
trustworthiness. Professionals know that good will can be
destroyed by a technically correct procedure in the best
medical interest of the patient which nonetheless offends
sentiments or raises questions about the medical value of
the procedure. While professionals deny patients the right
to form judgments on services, they know that patients do

form such judgments. Unfortunately, the argument that this
situation is alleviated by the adoption of a collectivity-orientation may mean only that careful image-management is
necessary to maintain medical credibility and the market
value of medical services. Theoretically, the requirements
for the maintenance of the medical relationship are satisfied
by the mere dramaturgical aspects of trust-inducement and
do not depend on the delivery of actual trustworthiness.

The considerations presented in this chapter have suggested a gap between Parsons' model of the institutionalization
of the medical profession and the actual institutionalization.
While practices theoretically necessary for good medical
services may correspond to the actual practices of the profession, the mere fact of correspondence does not adequately
explain institutionalization. While Parsons may believe that
functional considerations ought to be the driving force behind
the institutionalization of these practices, they need not be.
As will be seen in the following chapters, many of the
practices of the profession function in behalf of the collective
interests of the profession, whether or not they benefit the
patient in every instance. The institutionalization of the
profession, that is to say, does not require that the interests
of patients actually be met. At most, it requires only the
promise that these interests will be protected. In view of
the dramaturgical nature of maintaining "good will" in the
medical marketplace, in view of the randomness of ends to
which professional controls can be applied, in view of a
selective adaptation to the moral code by preferring situations of practice in which social controls are difficult if not
impossible to apply (such as in solo private practice), and in
view of components of the code which prevent the evaluative
process necessary for social control (such as the right of
privileged communication and the relegation of competence
to the sphere of personal conscience), whatever benefits
patients do receive by and large appear to be a function
of the physician's internalized sense of status honor and his
capacity for social understanding. These benefits are not
necessary for the existence of the profession, however much
Parsons might wish them to be.

I contend that Parsons' analysis of the profession through

professionalism, an ideological orientation, does not substantially explain the social phenomenon known in the United States and Britain as the medical profession. For one thing, the characteristic type of social organization that the profession has developed in not included in his definition. Parsons' theory of the professions follows from his desire to distinguish professionals from businessmen on the basis of their ideologically stated primary goal. This distinction echoes Max Weber's distinction between an economic group and a group with secondary economic interests. Weber's first type is organized on the basis of rationally controlled action which "may be oriented, in the actor's eyes, to purely economic results—want satisfaction or profit-making." His second type of group may use economic operations as a means for achieving different goals.[27] Weber's emphasis, however, was very different from Parsons'. Parsons' stress on the differences between professional and business ideologies with respect to ultimate goals stands in contrast to Weber's point that the differences between the two decrease in the face of economic and political determinants.

At some point economic conditions tend to become causally important, and often decisive, for almost all social groups, at least those which have major cultural significance; conversely, the economy is usually also influenced by the autonomous structure of social action within which it exists. No significant generalization can be made as to when and how this will occur. However, we can generalize about the degree of elective affinity between concrete structures of social action and concrete forms of economic organization; that means, we can state in general forms whether they are "adequate" or "inadequate" in relation to one another. We will have to deal frequently with such relations of adequacy. Moreover, at least some generalization can be advanced about the manner in which economic interests tend to result in social action of a certain type.[28]

[27] Max Weber, *Economy and Society: An Outline of Interpretive Sociology*, eds. Guenther Roth and Claus Wittich, 3 vols. (New York: Bedminster Press, 1968), p. 340.
[28] *Ibid.*, p. 341.

Groups that require large amounts of economic resources for the performance of ideal tasks will tend to adopt the same economic tactics as those oriented to the maximization of profit for personal sake, though they may adopt the same form of social organization under a different ideological rubric. The other side of the issue is that "primary economic groups" will tend to legitimize profitable gains by, among other means, the invocation of idealistic goals, including social utility.

In any event, the particular distinction necessary for understanding today's institutions is not that between professionalism and business ideologies. In the case of the medical profession, the most salient issue revolves around the distinction between professional versus bureaucratic social organization. Both can be ideologically oriented to a professionalism of the type Parsons characterizes as a collectivity-orientation, but the medical profession's insistence on retaining certain features characteristic of nonbureaucratic forms of social organization seems to be the real issue. Even Parsons has noted that certain practices in the medical profession are illogical from the point of view of professionalism. What he does not seem to appreciate is that arguments in defense of these practices are more than deviations from a pure ideology of professionalism; they are intended to preserve central institutions of the profession, not peripheral phenomena.

In conclusion, Parsons' theory of the medical profession is not a descriptive but a prescriptive theory which contains an explanatory theory of the institutionalization of the medical profession that is inadequate on a number of counts. It purports to explain the institutionalization of the profession in terms of the need for the social system to maintain healthy social actors to fulfill roles. While some roles may not be capable of being performed by the ill, Parsons does not adequately fill in the steps between this obvious observation and the creation of the medical profession. He does not, for instance, demonstrate that the activities of the medical profession are the major mechanism through which society sees to it that roles are fulfilled, and he does not demonstrate that the medical profession came about because of this "need" of the social system and not because of other considerations. Essentially, he does little more than assert that maintaining role systems would be harder without the activities of the medical profession (that is, the profession might not even be necessary—it just helps maintain the system) and then agrees that some of the profession's claims are logically consistent with this goal.

What is necessary is to consider a different approach to the problem of the institutionalization of the medical profession. Rather than focusing on the logical requirements for maintaining role systems, one may look at the political and economic requirements for the success of groups in society, trying thereby to explain the existence of the *group* which the profession is and leaving the relationship of this group to the rest of society open for analysis.

CHAPTER TWO

Toward an Adequate Theory of Institutionalization

What the current sociological literature lacks is an adequate theoretical understanding of professional institutionalization. The inadequacies of the Parsonian view of the profession require a fresh exploration of alternative approaches to the problem of institutionalization, and some consideration should be given to the general theoretical goals which any such theory should meet.

A comprehensive theory of institutionalization should specify at least the following: The types of social relationships which are institutionalized, the mechanisms, the agents, the facilitating conditions, and the driving forces of institutionalization. In a general sense, an explanation of institutionalization requires both ultimate and conditional reasons; that is, the driving forces behind institutionalization operate under specified conditions. One therefore cannot adequately account for concrete instances of institutionalization without answering such questions as the who, how, what, where, and when of the process.

The Weberian theory of economic action

An acceptable alternative approach to the problem of the institutional origins of the medical profession can be found

in Max Weber's *Economy and Society*. Weber's work did
not deal with this specific problem but was rather a more
ambitious attempt to investigate the institutional origins of
modern capitalism. Nonetheless, it suggests a number of
methodological and conceptual tools for dealing with this
problem.

Weber's mature work dealt with the problem of how a
particular type of economic group—modern capitalistic entrepreneurs—was successful under the conditions of modern
society. In *Economy and Society* he lays out the conceptual
framework necessary for tackling such an immensely complex problem.

According to Weber, virtually all groups engage in *economic action,* i.e., the satisfaction of wants for scarcities,
including the social relationships necessary for pursuing
satisfaction. Since most groups, even those without primary
economic goals, require scarcities to achieve their goals,
economic action is typically an important part of group life.[1]

Since economic action is a general feature of social life,
Weber investigated specific types of economic action: *economic conduct.* With this conceptual tool, he could address
the general question of the determinants of economic conduct, specifically of modern capitalism. As Weber noted in
his reaction to an essay by Rudolf Stammler, a broad but
"simple" distinction between the normative and empirical
aspects of economic action should be made. In this manner,
the determinants can be analyzed. The normative aspect is
the conception of what economic conduct should be, for
example, according to the legal theorist. The empirical or
sociological study of economic conduct examines the actual
reasons for why men engage in economic conduct. While
economic conduct may be in accordance with legal conceptions of proper economic conduct, one still does not know
the motives for compliance.[2]

The motives for empirical economic conduct are classified
into two broad categories: expediency (the pursuit of self-in-

[1] Max Weber, *Economy and Society: An Outline of Interpretive Sociology,* eds.
Guenther Roth and Claus Wittich, 3 vols. (New York: Bedminster Press, 1968),
pp. 339-341.
[2] *Ibid.,* pp. 32-33, 325-333.

terest) and legitimacy (the avoidance of negative sanctions).
As Weber formulated this:

> . . . economic action . . . is oriented to knowledge of
> the relative scarcity of certain available means to want
> satisfaction, in relation to the actor's state of needs and
> to the present and probable action of others, insofar as
> the latter affects the same resources. But at the same
> time, of course, the actor in his choice of economic
> procedures naturally orients himself *in addition* to the
> conventional and legal rules which he recognizes as valid,
> that is, of which he knows that a violation on his part
> would call forth a given reaction of other persons.[3]

Weber expanded this conception of the motives of empirical
economic action to include habit (simply doing what one
always has done, without calculation of outcomes), expediency (calculation of the effect of outcomes on self-interest),
and legitimacy (acting out of a sense of obligation or duty,
even in the face of conflicting self-interest). Legitimacy
includes behavior performed on account of custom, convention, or law, that is, behavior oriented to certain bodies of
belief, which is categorized according to method of enforcement. "Custom," for example, is a norm which simply carries
the weight of the past to influence behavior. A "convention,"
however, is a norm which when violated brings about social
disapproval. A "law" is a norm which, even if carrying the
weight of the past and bringing about social disapproval,
also has an organized, specialized staff ready and disposed
to enforce it with various coercive means. Insofar as legitimacy enters in as a motive for economic action, these
institutionally specific norms are determinants of economic
conduct, yet Weber never meant them as the sole determinants of economic conduct. Instead, they modulate action
which is conducted on the basis of self-interest.[4]

Because economic action is directed toward the acquisition
of scarcities, Weber noted, groups tend to become conflict
groups, which may engage in violent or peaceful conflict,
depending on the application of physical force. Regulated

[3] *Ibid.*, p. 33.
[4] *Ibid.*, pp. 29-38, 311, 325.

peaceful conflict is competition. While violent conflict may well be a determinant of the success of certain groups, competition may be an equally significant determinant and more susceptible to analytical treatment. Weber apparently meant in this instance that although empirical economic action requires explanation in terms of motives, the historical success of specific types of economic conduct requires explanation in terms of "the conditions in which the conflict or competition takes place. . . . *Among* the decisive conditions, it must not be forgotten, belong the systems of order to which the behavior of parties is oriented, whether traditionally, as a matter of rationally disinterested loyalty *(wertrational)*, or of expediency."[5] By the social selection of individuals with qualities compatible with the conditions of conflict, certain types of behavior become successful.[6]

Groups can to an extent alter their qualities to increase their chances of success under given conditions of conflict. One method of doing so is to vary the size of membership, to restrict or expand it depending on the group's situation. Though expansion simply requires opening participation to whomever wishes it and engaging in tactics to attract new members, restriction requires the capacity to deny membership to some who wish it. Restriction, or monopolization, then is a dominative as well as economic process inasmuch as the group attempts to interfere with the will of others.[7]

Weber distinguished between power (the capacity to carry out one's *own* will despite resistance) and domination (the capacity to get *others* to carry out one's will). Insofar as monopolization is a requirement for group success, domination becomes a requirement for group success. Domination, like economic action, has normative and empirical aspects. The normative aspect of domination is authority, or the right to obtain compliance with commands; yet actual domination can occur on illegitimate or nonlegitimate grounds as well, and authority can contribute to actual domination. The distinction can adequately be handled by a distinction between authoritative and de facto types of empirical domina-

[5] *Ibid.*, p. 39.
[6] *Ibid.*, pp. 38-40.
[7] *Ibid.*, p. 43.

tion. Authoritative domination takes place on the basis of claims of legitimate command; de facto domination takes place on the basis of favorable constellations of interest between superordinate and subordinate figures.[8] As in the analysis of types of legitimate economic conduct, authoritative domination can be subdivided into customary, conventional, and legal domination, depending on the type of enforcement likely to be mobilized in behalf of issued commands.

Domination, however, is a feature of both a group's adaptive capacity and the conditions of conflict. Particularly groups which compete under the regulative domination of a political community (a structure of domination over a territory) such as the state (a political community which commands a monopoly on the use of physical force) are subordinate parties in the dominative relationship.[9] Political domination, therefore, becomes a major determinant of the outcome of group competition under such historical conditions.

The success of a group, therefore, is a function of two broad determinants of economic action: The group's tactics of competition (or of conflict) and the conditions of competition. One major but not exclusive condition of competition in modern society is the state, which exercises both authoritative and de facto domination over groups within its territory. Since the body of norms for which the state acts as an enforcement staff is the legal order, politically oriented action by competitive groups must take into account the constraining effects of law and the competitive advantages of being able to influence legislation.

The Weberian theory of monopolization

Weber's theory of monopolization is particularly pertinent to the problem of the institutionalization of the medical

---

[8] Cf. the succinct note by Guenther Roth on Weber, *op. cit.*, pp. 61-62, for a discussion of the problems of translating *Herrschaft*. "Domination" refers to compliance with the commands of a staff which employs both legitimacy and force to secure compliance. I have simply invented phrases to help keep distinct the various implications of the term *Herrschaft*.

[9] *Ibid.*, p. 54.

profession, because it helps explain how the organizational conduct of groups can increase their adaptive capacity and chances for success. In this respect, it suggests a mechanism for the institutionalization of the medical profession. To be sure, monopolization is not the only mechanism for group success. Expansion of membership can also contribute to group success under appropriate conditions. Yet the history of the medical profession seems to me to have been marked more by monopolization activities than by expansionism, and I shall concentrate my analytical efforts on the monopolization aspects of the profession's success.

The central significance of Weber's theory of monopolization lies in its analysis of the manner in which group organization is able to help individuals further their interests. As the number of competitors within an activity encroaches upon the profit span, an interest is created in the exclusion of some competitors. Concerted action in behalf of closure may take the form of mere joint action, the formation of associational groups such as guilds, and the acquisition of legal privileges from the political community. Apparently the most efficacious means of closure is for the associational group to persuade the legitimate agents of force within a political community to recognize and enforce the group's monopolistic claims. It then becomes what Weber calls a legally privileged group, a group with a legal privilege to hold a monopoly. Regulation of closure may be based on either exclusion on the basis of some readily identifiable characteristics of external competitors—such as "race, language, religion, local or social origins, descent, residence, etc."[10]—or inclusion on the basis of some qualities "acquired through upbringing, apprenticeship, and training."[11] In Weber's terminology, a distinction is made between the types of associational action on the basis of the method of regulation of closure. Therefore, a restrictive association based on the exclusion of outsiders is an interest group, and one based on the inclusion of insiders with particular acquired characteristics is a guild.

Intrusion upon a profit span is not the only motive for

[10] *Ibid.*, p. 342.
[11] *Ibid.*, p. 344.

monopolization. Men may join together in concerted action to further one another's interests in any competitive situation. These interests may be either primarily economic or ideal; nonetheless, there is a tendency toward some degree of monopolistic action in either event, since ideal missions tend to require economic resources for success. This requirement for material resources tends to replace an orientation toward ideal goals with a concern for the preservation of the interest group. Therefore, Weber notes that in the case of many groups with acquired skills, though an interest in guaranteeing efficient performance may have some motivational importance in monopolization, "normally this concern for efficient performance recedes behind the interest in limiting the supply of candidates for the benefices and honors of a given occupation.[12]

More generally, "interest in the substance of the shared ideals" of a primarily noneconomic group (usually a secondary economic group) "necessarily recedes behind the interest in the persistence or propaganda of the group.[13] Preservation of the group can be attained by the creation and possession of scarcities, and so the group tends to lay exclusive claim on valued material and human objects and to restrict membership in the group. To the degree that the group successfully increases the attributes that bring wealth and prestige through the monopolization of scarcities, men who are attracted to these secondary goals more than the ideals find their way into the group. Monopolization therefore expands the number of men who wish to join the group. Therefore, even secondary economic groups then face the problem of restricting group entry. Typically an attempt is made to exclude outsiders from the group and even insiders from certain internal positions.[14]

As Weber's brilliant analysis suggests, monopolization requires domination over the market in order to exclude competitors from a group. To this extent the study of monopolization is the study of domination by social groups

[12] *Ibid.*
[13] *Ibid.*, p. 345.
[14] *Ibid.*, pp. 43-46, 341-348.

over the market. Such domination is usually a mixture of domination on the basis of constellations of interests (de facto domination) and on the basis of formally acquired (often legal) authority (authoritative domination). Indeed, the term "monopolization" refers as much to the domination required for closure as to the closure proper. For this reason, the Weberian usage is not a narrowly economic meaning.

The applicability of the Weberian theory of monopolization for the study of the institutionalization of the medical profession

Weber classifies the medical profession as a type of commercial class. Professionals constitute a class insofar as they share common economic interests on the basis of their market situation, which in their case is determined by the marketability of services. Positively privileged commercial classes, which include merchants, shipowners, bankers and financiers, along with "professionals with sought-after expertise or privileged education (such as lawyers, physicians, artists)," consist of potentially competitive entrepreneurs. Because of this latent competition, concerted action in behalf of common interests need not arise merely on the basis of a common class situation.[15] That it does arise, as in the formation of guilds, requires explanation.

It is the development of class organizations from the commercial class of professionals which is best explained by the theory of monopolization. While some measure of intragroup competition may still be permitted by a monopolistic organization, the competitive advantages of monopolization by organized groups help explain the formation and structure of organized professional groups. I am interested, then, in the creation of guild-type organizations among medical professionals as instruments of the profession's collective interests, and secondarily in the effects of such organization on the relationships between medical professionals and their patients.

Medical professionals have formed a variety of guild-type organizations and have developed a variety of tactics for

[15] *Ibid.*, pp. 302-304.

domination in behalf of monopolization. This is consistent with the predominantly peaceful type of conflict in which professionals engage. They have constructed most of the rules for the regulation of economic conduct on the part of professionals, which Weber notes is nearly a pure type of autonomous organization.[16] Furthermore, they have established varying degrees of domination over both the modern market and modern legislative institutions of the state.

In several respects, the history of the medical profession illustrates the appropriateness of Weber's theory of monopolization, particularly with regard to monopolization as a form of both domination and rational economic conduct. Ten of the many aspects of the general process of monopolization seem to stand out on the basis of the historical studies which are to follow:

1. The creation of commodities. In most cases of economic exchange involving goods or raw materials, there is little question about what is for sale. In the case of the professions, services are offered for sale. Services are not, however, tangible items and so require a certain amount of persuasion to convert them into commodities. Their creation is an important aspect of monopolization insofar as they are prerequisites for domination over the market. The task is to convince a buyer that the service is a commodity, that it should be sold for a price or fee, and that other forms of exchange such as friendship are not legitimate. The American Medical Association, one of the guild-type class organizations of the medical profession, has frequently preferred that patients pay for services whenever possible as a matter of moral principle and has tended to reject alternative payment methods.

2. The separation of the performance of services from the satisfaction of client interests. In the medical profession it is also important to separate the commodity creation of services from meliorative results. Economic interests are favored by the capacity to sell medical services, for example, without having to guarantee a "cure." This separation creates a larger body of salable services. Even "services"

[16] *Ibid.*, pp. 49-50.

which do not improve patient health can be charged for; a service becomes redefined as an act in which certain skills are applied to a problem rather than an act which increases the life-condition or life-chances of the patient.

3. The creation of scarcity. This can be achieved either through decreasing supply by reducing the availability of a commodity or through increasing demand by upgrading the quality of the commodity to increase marginal utility. In the case of the medical profession, scarcity has been most effectively achieved by both reducing supply and increasing demand through the same institutional mechanism: licensing. By setting high standards for licensure, higher quality services can be claimed, the marginal utility of services increased, and the proportion of qualified suppliers reduced through strict licensing requirements.

4. The monopolization of supply. A monopolistic group seeks to secure sole supply in the market through three means: uniting individual suppliers, driving competitive suppliers out of the market by using various economic tactics, and persuading the state to eliminate competitors by preferential legal treatment. Of these three, legal privilege has been most effective in the case of the profession. The mere unification of individual suppliers does not create scarcity because of limitations on the amount of services individual practitioners can afford to withhold from the market, and because of the necessity for practitioners to be willing to withhold them. Driving competitors from the market is difficult in the case of services, since ownership of the inputs of production is not as critical as with tangible goods, and more complex mechanisms are necessary to control these inputs. Exclusion has been achieved in the market in general only when the inputs of commodity production have first been monopolized by a single supplier. In the professions, the task has been to monopolize education, which is analogous to input factors in the manufacture of goods. This relationship illuminates the interest that practicing medical professionals have had in dominating institutions of professional education. The monopolization of education, however, is difficult: in a field where competence is uncertain, many can claim

to possess proper education and, if enterprising enough, can go on to open medical schools. Such has in fact happened wherever the political community has not established a legal system of licensure superordinate to diplomas. Therefore, typically the creation of a monopoly on supply requires some measure of preferential legal treatment at the points of both supply and production.

5. Restriction of group membership. Closure is the chief means for making services scarce and a necessary condition for the formation of a monopolistic group. Restriction serves the interests of the group's members in three ways. It increases membership loyalty by increasing per capita income within the same market, independently raises prices by decreasing supply relative to demand, and helps make possible noncompetitive relationships among group members, a matter which will be discussed shortly.

6. The elimination of external competition. Following the creation of a monopolistic group through membership restriction, it is in the interest of the group to eliminate competitive sources of supply. Typically, the group claims to supply the only authentic commodity (e.g., declares others "quacks") and makes a variety of efforts to put its competitors out of business. Even a legally privileged group must still see to it that favorable laws are enforced. If not a legally privileged group, it may try to eliminate competition by producing a more marketable commodity by directly preventing competitors from making their supply available on the market. For a variety of reasons, preventing competitors from making their supply available is virtually impossible without two strategies which have historically been used by the medical profession: ethical claims to raise the marginal utility of the group's services, and legal licensure to bring the force and prestige of the political community to bear against competitors. These strategies are by no means mutually exclusive; the medical profession in the United States, for example, has employed both methods. Of the two, legal licensure is more reliable than popular recognition, for it requires less widespread acceptance of the validity of legitimacy claims to eliminate external competitors.

7. The capacity to fix prices above theoretical competitive market value. The price of services is not a "natural" value but is determined by the workings of the marketplace. Under certain circumstances, price is determined by the classical forces of supply and demand; but when competition is suppressed, prices can be independently determined. Buyers can boycott to bring down prices, and suppliers can agree among themselves to sell at a fixed price without regard for fluctuations in demand. It is in the interest of group members to reject competitive pricing in favor of price fixing in order to maximize total group income. Where competition has been suppressed and price fixing established, price limits still exist in the sense that it is not economically rational to price services out of the market; that is, there is a price which optimally maximizes total group profits. Since restriction of membership is an alternative means for raising prices, extreme restriction can theoretically also bring prices up to the same optimum price as price fixing. But short of such extreme restriction, price fixing remains the most effective means for optimizing group income. Before 1912, the American medical profession attempted formal price fixing by including uniform fees in its official codes of medical ethics and calling for adherence to medical society fee tables. Price fixing, however, need not be formal. Even where prohibited by antimonopolistic or antitrust legislation, as in the United States, price fixing can still be accomplished through customary or traditional fee scales for professional services. Even though an individual professional is free to charge what he pleases, his desire to charge a "fair fee" may take the form of charging approximately the same as his colleagues, and so uniformity tends to occur, though not through competitive pricing mechanisms. Price fixing recast in moral terms remains price fixing.

8. The unification of suppliers. Because control over the sale of services is not in the hands of any single person, the members of a monopolistic service group are economically rational if they behave as though they were collectively a single supplier. Coordination requires the development of a sense of mutual interests, group identification, and the cre-

ation of a system of group controls to ensure equal pricing. The temptation to set prices on an individual basis, particularly the temptation of immediate gain, threatens the maintenance of action in behalf of group interests. The individualizing tendencies of economic interests therefore require a certain measure of balance by appeals to integrative economic rationality, moral duty, technical rationality, or by coercive means in the form of ostracism or expulsion. Because members are differentially sensitive to long-range economic appeals, status appeals may well be substituted. Competitive economic behavior may therefore be ironically denounced as material acquisitiveness, even though in reality noncompetition may result in greater long-range gain for all members.

9. The elimination of internal competition. The organizational principle that economic competition prevents successful price fixing leads to efforts among group members to curtail intragroup competition. The usual mechanism by which professional intragroup competition has been discouraged has been medical ethics; certain economic practices such as price competition, advertising and bargaining have been strongly condemned and can be submitted as grounds for expulsion from medical soceties and even for legal revocation of a license to practice. All forms of competition for patients, not only price competition, have typically been prohibited as well.

10. The development of group solidarity and cooperativeness. Fraternalistic devices constitute some of the major noneconomic means by which internal competition is eliminated. Weber refers to these qualities as the communal relationship present in all associational relationships, i.e., the nonrational sentiments which can integrate a group beyond that which is made possible by rational calculation. These are advantageous to the group in several ways. They help prevent competition by discouraging the eruption of latent conflicts among members. They provide subjective rewards of participation sociability. They predispose members to protect one another's interests in the face of outside attacks on members or the group as a whole. And they encourage

arrangements among members that help each other obtain buyers in the event that a system of differentiated supply exists within the group, such as a specialist referral system. Most important, they help make members interested in furthering the collective interests of the group and not merely their own personal interests. Such fraternalistic devices are commonplace in the medical profession, as in the cases of the provision of free medical care to fellow practitioners and the tendency of practitioners to defend one another against criticism.

The monopolistic features of the medical profession mentioned above require a certain measure of group domination for success. To be sure, monopolization can facilitate domination, but for now I will confine my discussion to the dominative requirements of monopolization. The organized medical profession has sought domination over others as well as the freedom to carry out its own will. Indeed, the profession has tended to determine both its own and others' goals with respect to medical issues.

The dominative character of much of medical professional life cannot be underestimated. Even the technical goals of the profession are dominative: physicians may wish to be free to act as they think best, but they also expect their patients to adhere to their advice. The physician claims authority to define the patient's interests and to select the means for achieving them, and the patient is expected to comply. Parallel with technical interests are the social and economic concerns of the profession, which also have dominative aspects. A physician's legal right to set and collect fees is a form of domination which the free laborer has not acquired. The physician as a professional, unlike the free laborer, is in a position to command his employer, though he can only hope for compliance in the absence of any staff to enforce commands. In the absence of compliance, the physician does not have economic sanctions to exercise against the patient, because he is the patient's employee; he usually can only appeal to the patient's self-protective interests, or in special cases, can obtain court orders and apply physical coercion.

Yet to an extent, the dominative relationship is a reversal of normal employer-employee relations. The free laborer is employed on the condition that he follow his employer's commands or risk being dismissed, while the professional claims the right in the relationship to issue commands or instructions and the right to disregard the patient's instructions if he thinks best. Even the professional who disregards his employer's instructions is still usually able to claim payment under the law, which the free laborer cannot. Indeed, one of the most important legal contributions to the dominative position of the medical profession accompanied licensure provisions in English-speaking nations prior to the last half of the nineteenth century: the right to sue for fees. True, even unlicensed professionals had the right to set fees in contrast to the employer's right to declare the terms of a wage contract with a free laborer, but only licensed practitioners could bring to bear the enforcement mechanisms of the political community against those who would not pay fees. These considerations of domination, then, have been important institutional features in the development of the profession as a group, both as sources of success for the profession and as means for distinguishing the professions from other groups in society.

Patients, moreover, have not been the only social group over which organized professionals have attempted to establish domination. Other objects of domination have included the medical schools, both within and independent of universities, hospitals, auxiliary health personnel, and the state in its various structural manifestations. In America, for instance, medical schools have been dominated at least by the right of accreditation jointly claimed by the practitioner-based American Medical Association and the academic-based American Association of Medical Colleges. No school, in fact, can be accredited without AMA approval, a right, which, as will be seen subsequently, has important consequences in view of the fact that most licensing boards are controlled wholly or in part by representatives of the state medical societies affiliated with the AMA; through control of licensing boards the AMA's accreditation of medical schools is given legal force, and through this network of controls the curriculum of medical schools and even the number of schools have been to a large extent determined. Until recently, a staff appointment in a hospital had been very difficult to obtain even for graduates of AMA-accredited schools who were not members of medical societies. Hospitals, too, have been subject to accreditation proceedings by the AMA. Hospital personnel, such as nurses, have long been held subordinate to the commands of doctors, and on an organizational level, the professional aspirations of "paraprofessionals" have been checked by the refusal of the medical profession's representatives to surrender control in certain areas. The state, for good measure, has been extremely reluctant to act in matters regarding health care except upon the advice of the AMA's counsel. The AMA, perhaps, has not wielded total domination over these groups and institutions; the federal government, for example, has refused to implement certain AMA policies such as an independent cabinet-level Health Department. Yet the government is committed to recognizing the authority of the medical profession in matters of practice and has had considerable difficulty in determining where the limits of professional authority lie.

The structure of the medical profession

Inasmuch as the structure of the medical profession as a form of class organization has tended to approximate Weber's type of the guild, certain details of this structure can be specified by comparing the organizational forms which the medical profession has typically assumed with the type of the bureaucracy which Weber has outlined in *Economy and Society*.

Before beginning the technical discussion, I offer a caveat. The bureaucratization of practitioners is not the same as the bureaucratization of the practice setting. Bureaucratization of the work setting refers to the development of bureaucratized administrative settings such as hospitals, the military, and other such organized settings in which doctors may work. Yet the fact that the doctor must deal with bureaucratized laymen in the course of his practice does not mean that doctors themselves become bureaucratized with respect to one another. Indeed, doctors typically do not establish domination over one another, except perhaps in specialized settings such as training hospitals. The organizational problem of the bureaucratization of the practitioner, i.e., of the relationship of practitioners to one another, is a separate concern, and one bearing a need for investigation.

For a technical definition of bureaucratization, the classical one is the type of bureaucracy described by Weber, which is characterized by a number of principles. The first is. the principle of *official jurisdictional areas* ordered by rules. These jurisdictional areas specify official duties for their incumbents, and authority is stably distributed in accordance with them, delimited by rules concerning legitimate coercive means. These official duties are regularly and continuously fulfilled only by qualified persons. There is also the principle of *office hierarchy* and channels of appeal, in which lower offices are supervised by higher offices. This hierarchy is monocratic in the extreme case, and it may be dominated by either private or public authority. Office management in bureaucracy is based on preserved written documents. There is *segregation of official activity from the sphere of private life* in two senses. Public resources or business assets—the means of administration or service—are not owned by the official; they are divorced from his private property. And the authority of the official is based on the authority inherent in his office, not his person. This divorce of authority from the person derives from the existence of official jurisdictional areas along which authority is distributed. Office management is also based on thorough training in a field of specialization. Such training is more necessary for highly specialized duties. Furthermore, the full working capacity of the official is required, irrespective of length of obligatory working hours. The official's duty is to work at full capacity despite the absence of economic incentives due to salaried employment. Also, office management follows general rules, which themselves come to represent specialized technical expertise. Thus, there is created a staff of offices oriented to impersonal and functional purposes. Where the need for expert services is high, the social esteem of the office is high, and can be enjoyed by the officeholder. Economic rewards are in the form of monetary salaries usually fixed according to the status of the office held. While it would be most logical for the maximization of impersonal goals to appoint officials on the basis of technical expertise, the career interests of officials moving between hierarchical positions within the bureaucracy tend to favor the development of promotion on the basis of seniority. Ideally, however, *promotion should be on the basis of task competence.*[17]

Professionalization of practitioners contrasts with the idea of the bureaucracy at several points. There is a *general absence of jurisdictional areas.* Authority to perform certain duties is delegated uniformly on the basis of the possession of a license to practice and not according to a system of offices. This idea is embodied in the ideal of the general practitioner, who is legally permitted to perform any medical task not specifically proscribed by law. While some degree of task differentiation may arise in the form of specialists, the existence of specialists does not exclude generalists from practicing in specialty areas. *Specialization threatens professionalization* to the extent that specialists might break away to form separate monopolistic groups and restrict practice in specialty areas to specialists, or even without breaking away, might generate competition between specialists and generalists for patients.

There is also a *general absence of formal hierarchization.* Not only are offices absent, but there is a fraternal egalitarian quality to the relationships of practitioners to one another. This aspect has several consequences. Problems of coordination of specialized services tend to be ignored because of reluctance to establish hierarchical relationships of authority necessary for coordination. Differences among practitioners in competence in certain areas also tend to be ignored due to a reluctance to establish supervision over work performance. Informal hierarchization occurs, however, on the basis of status distinctions in the form of "reputation" and other potentially nontechnical, nonobjective criteria. Rewards tend to be awarded on an equal basis for all members of

[17] *Ibid.*, pp. 956-963.

the profession rather than being graduated along hierarchical lines.

Professionalization tends to *associate professional and private life*. Professionals typically own their means of practice (their equipment) whenever possible, in order to avoid dependence on others and the assumption of supervisory positions by others. Authority to perform certain tasks is a function of the personal possession of a license and does not require appointment to an office. And unlike bureaucrats, the performance of services by professionals directly affects their economic rewards. That is, they collect fees on the basis of specific services rather than salaries.

Even more important than the means of remuneration for services is the *absence of a system of promotion* under professionalization. The lack of an office hierarchy eliminates the possibility of rewarding demonstrated competence with promotion to a higher official status and salary position. Indeed, it is difficult to structure economic rewards under professionalization in order to encourage quality technical work, due the income-leveling tendencies of professionalization. On the other hand, it is not as necessary to include demands for full capacity work under professionalization, due to the work-encouraging nature of the fee-for-service structure.

In some respects, professionalization is similar to bureaucratization. Preserved written records are common to both, even though they play a larger role in official interaction among members of a bureaucracy. Both demand full working capacity and see work as a full-time vocation rather than an avocation. Both enjoy high social esteem, due to the nature of the expert services provided, and most important of all, both are oriented toward an impersonal functional purpose and not merely the satisfaction of private interests. Due to the hierarchical nature of bureaucratization, however, the bureaucrat is less likely to participate in policy making, that is, in the determination of the goals of action, and so his private interests are less likely to shape policies. This is not to say that someone's private interests will not shape policies, but the bureaucrat is far less likely to make his private interests felt than is the relatively independent individual member of a profession.

Though Weber's ideal type of the bureaucracy helps us clarify a definition of the profession through detailed contrasts, one should still allow for the development of multiple types which the profession has historically assumed. The profession has developed in different ways in various social and historical settings, and to provide a more adequate account of what has been institutionalized, one should be able to specify which types the profession has elaborated and, ideally, identify crucial factors which have led to the ascendancy of one or another type. The investigation of these types of professional organization will be one of the major tasks of examining the medical profession in concrete settings.

The conditions of competition

So far I have considered four of the requirements of a comprehensive theory of group institutionalization. I have specified the types of social relationships which have tended to be institutionalized by the medical profession, the mechanisms by which they are established (monopolization), the agents of institutionalization (members of the organized conflict group which constitutes or at least dominates the medical profession), and the driving forces behind institutionalization (the attempt to satisfy the wants of group members). The appropriate conditions for institutionalization have received little attention, though Weber has at least pointed attention in certain directions.

Weber's distinction between action on the basis of expediency versus action on the basis of fear of enforcement led to a theoretical discussion of the legitimacy of certain cultural systems of norms as the objects of enforcement. Within this context, legitimacy is significant as a *constraint* on expedient action. By the same token, I would offer, legitimacy as a constraint is one of the conveniently analyzable conditions of competition (i.e., regulated conflict). Since the medical profession as a monopolistic body of practitioners has arisen within a political community, I am particularly

interested in the role of the legal order as a constraint on
the medical profession's group success.

Yet even the legal order as a system of constraints can
provide appropriate conditions for successful group monopolization. The conversion of an interest group into a legally
privileged group is one such instance of selective advantage.

The phenomenon of legal privilege begs the question,
however, of which conditions led to the bestowal of legal
privileges. Weber did not address this question systematically, since he was more interested in the social consequences
of the tendency of groups to monopolize than in the factors
which make certain groups more successful than others. Yet
scattered throughout his work are examples of how this
question might be answered. I shall return to these examples
in a later chapter, when their discussion will be more appropriate. For now, I can provisionally divide this problem of
the conditions of competition into two major parts: (a) what
factors conduce men to pursue their interests in groups rather
than as individuals? That is, which conditions favor the
formation of conflict groups? (b) what factors facilitate the
rise of monopolies?

In the following chapters, I intend to apply Weber's theory
of monopolization, not to refute it. I will examine three
phenomena: medical ethics, licensure in England and the
United States, and a medical care reorganization proposal.
I will demonstrate the appropriateness of Weber's theory
of monopolization but will also use the substantive materials
to specify some of the issues discussed in this chapter, such
as the types of social relationships which the medical profession has tended to assume and the conditions of competition
which have selected the organized medical profession for
success.

CHAPTER THREE

Medical Ethics and Monopolization

As norms dictating proper conduct for doctors, medical ethics provide material for analyzing the official ideals of the relationships doctors are expected to achieve. Since medical ethics have changed throughout history, they can also serve as aids for the analysis of changes in the structure of the profession and of the relationship of the profession to larger society. Medical ethics are most interesting, however, because of their role as organizational tools or resources in the institutionalization of the profession as a social group, particularly with their role as components of professional monopolization.

While a full account of the origins of medical ethics in terms of the experiences which led to the formulation of specific ethical provisions would be valuable, information on this level about the origins of ethics remains unavailable for the vast majority of ethical systems. Modern historians are fortunate to possess even the present incomplete record of ancient codes. Such an analysis is not necessary, however, if medical ethics are understood as more than cultural phenomena. Ethics are sociologically important as a contribution to the organization of the profession, and not merely as ends in themselves.

A survey of medical ethics reveals a remarkable amount of variation throughout history. The Hippocratic ethics, the oldest known system of medical ethics, probably dates back more than 2000 years, and since then systems of medical ethics not sharing Hippocratic attitudes have periodically appeared. When one considers medical ethics, one must consider medieval ethics, Enlightenment ethics, and official codes of ethics promulgated by modern medical practitioner associations. In doing so, one will find that these ethical systems possess varying degrees of organizational utility and, indeed, that they can serve several types of organizational uses. Historical variation, then, suggests that perhaps the organizational strategies of the medical profession have changed and so one might consider two general questions: (1) How can ethics become conducive to group interest pursuit, i.e., the organizational strategies of the profession and the organizational theories on which they have been based? and (2) What are the reasons for changes in ethical codes? While one might consider either of these questions solely from the point of view of the profession as a group, I suggest that the nature of larger society changes and the profession changes accordingly. So, ethical codes may change as the profession devises more efficient and effective means for achieving its organizational goals, but they may also change because the group's political (external) requirements change.

The conversion of medical ethics into political and organizational tools can assume at least three forms of politicization: innovative, revisionary, and confrontational. Innovative politicization is the de novo creation of politically favorable ethical provisions. One example is the appearance in the 1949 "Principles of Ethics" of the American Medical Association of a prohibition against providing professional services to any agency which profits by them. This innovation occurred in response to the development of third-party arrangements, some of which might have threatened the traditional organization of private physicians. Revisionary politicization is the creation of specific exceptions to preexisting ethical rules. The 1912 "Principles of Ethics" of the American Medical Association, for instance, permitted breaking the ancient rule of professional secrecy whenever required by the law or public health considerations. Revision occurs when it seems more prudent to yield to political exigencies rather than to confront them. Confrontational politicization, by contrast, is the application of preexisting ethical rules to emergent political purposes. Professional secrecy, for instance, is a prebureaucratic ethical rule which has been subsequently invoked in opposition to certain bureaucratizing proposals in recent decades. While not created as an obstacle to bureaucratization, it has acquired new value in the struggle between the profession and forces which might dominate the profession, for it forbids evaluation by outsiders.

As I have suggested, ethics can become politicized, but they can acquire new political functions as well. Because sequential codes face up to organizational problems which may not have affected preexisting codes, each code gives the appearance of a change of phase as one problem after another is tackled. Some codes integrate physicians into an interest group and reduce internal competition; others eliminate external competition; others build cordial relations with political authorities and legislators; others adapt to new legal restraints; and still others build favorable public opinion. I think it valuable, then, to see how medical ethics have correspondingly changed with the changing political position of the medical profession and have helped direct the profession's political development.

To conduct these studies, one need not engage in a moral analysis of the medical profession. I do not intend to judge the value of medical ethics for medical care but wish to examine the causal role which ethics have played in the profession's institutionalization. Recognizing tendencies toward politicization, for instance, need not imply cynicism in the guise of scientific scholarship. Politically useful ethics may still have value for effective medical care and reflect the moral sincerity of professionals. Ethics are not mere superstructures or hypocritical rationalizations for interest pursuit but an integral part in the organization of the profession.

Ethics are a special organizational tool: appeals to men with self-identities of being highly principled, who tend to give little attention to the institutionalization problems of the profession because of busy everyday schedules. They are a means for achieving political effectiveness as a group without requiring *Realpolitik* consciousness from rank-and-file members. Ethics in fact tend to decrease political awareness among most professionals by confounding consequences with morals; they permit justifying decisions by simple labelling as "ethical," thereby shutting off contemplation and discussion. So politicized ethics can be interpreted as evidence of the profession's moral sincerity just as well as of conspiratorial cynicism. Similarly, recognizing the political components of ethics can be consistent with relative objectivity on the part of the social observer as well as with possible cynicism.

Nor is the examination of the consequences of ethics for institutionalization a single motif argument. Ethics need not be compatible with favorable institutionalization. The concept of politicization even implies some freedom as well as interplay between the development of medical ethics and the institutionalization of the profession. Since not all systems of ethics have favored the profession's group development and success, the question arises of which social theories were necessary for professional institutionalization.

Certain medical ethical problems will not be a part of the following discussion. Current ethical discussions about permissible procedures, therapeutic experimentation, informed consent, reactions to death, the definition of time of death, and a larger series of issues about research in medicine have not yet been incorporated into official codes of ethics and may never be. As attempts to structure norms for these problems, they are extremely important discussions and will likely have a long-range effect on future medical practice. Their political relevance, however, is not as clear; and so I decline to discuss them.

The first section to follow will analyze Thomas Percival's much respected 1803 *Medical Ethics,* a work of the English medical profession. I will use Weber's theory of monopolization to suggest how ethics might have been used to help the profession pursue collective interests. I will also investi-

gate the manner in which the profession's political setting
influenced the structure of ethics, that is, the political uses
of Percival's ethics. Percival's ethics, while not as politicized
as some later codes, provide numerous initial insights into
causal relationships. The second section will examine the
implicit assumptions of social theory contained in several
systems of ethics, beginning with the work of Hippocrates.
It will help clarify the ethical changes required for interest-
group formation and will demonstrate how some ethical
systems fell into disfavor because of the changing political
conditions of the profession. The third section will study
the vicissitudes of the American Medical Association's code
of ethics. These vicissitudes suggest changes in the profession's political setting and the profession's response. A fourth
section will compare the relationship of different systems
of ethics to institutionalization requirements on specific
issues: the concept of medical service, fee setting, the role
of the political arm of the profession, and the relative merits
of ethics and licensure as mechanisms of monopolization.
Through these studies, a clearer understanding of the organization of professionals and of the profession's relationship
to society will be achieved.

Percivalean ethics and monopolization

Thomas Percival (1740-1804) is best remembered as the
foremost spokesman for the conservative wing of the medical
Enlightenment in England by virtue of his *Medical Ethics,*
written in 1794 and published in 1803. Born in England, he
entered the great medical school at Edinburgh and received
his M.D. from Leyden in 1765. That year, he was also made
a Fellow of the Royal Society and settled in Manchester
to practice. Well known for his social and philosophical work,
he corresponded regularly with Franklin, Voltaire, Diderot
and D'Alembert. In 1791, he was asked by the medical staff
of the Manchester Infirmary "to draw up a scheme of
professional conduct relative to hospitals and other medical

charities,"[1] following a dispute among house staff in 1789 that had led to resignations. Percival had close friends on both sides in the dispute, and his work apparently had some conciliatory effect. The code itself consisted of four sections: "Of Professional Conduct, Relative to Hospitals, or Other Medical Charities," "Of Professional Conduct in Private or General Practice," "Of the Conduct of Physicians Towards Apothecaries," and "Of Professional Duties, in Certain Cases which Require a Knowledge of Law." I will deal only with the section on private or general practice, for it was on the basis of this section that half a century later the newly founded American Medical Association constructed its own "Code of Medical Ethics" and claimed continuity with Percival's famous work.

Percival's section on general practice contains advice in six areas: trust building, consultations among physicians, taking over another physician's patient, economic policy, promoting the honor and interests of the profession, retrospection, and miscellany. His advice in each area will first be reviewed and then its role in the profession's institutionalization examined, particularly its role in monopolization.

The bulk of Percival's trust-building prescriptions are general moral rules of conduct: attention, steadiness, humanity, secrecy, delicacy, and confidence. Others pertain to the physician's quality of mind: temperance for the sake of clear thought, and retirement when senility sets in. Others have to do more specifically with handling the patient: reasonable numbers of visits to the sick, not abandoning doomed patients, admonitions to patients suffering from the wages of sin, observance of the Sabbath for both themselves and the patient except in emergencies, and abstention from gloomy prognostications to maintain hope and comfort in the sick except when the patient must make his own death arrangements.[2]

[1] Chauncey D. Leake, ed., *Percival's Medical Ethics* (Baltimore: Williams & Wilkins, 1927), p. 31.

[2] *Ibid.*, sections I-III, XIII, XXIX-XXXII, pp. 90-91, 97-98, 107-111.

Such trust-inducing devices bear specific relationships to monopolization. In a general way, trust inducement increases the market value of medical services and helps convert them into commodities. Similarly, it flatters doctors and helps integrate them into a professional group, thereby furthering group formation. It also creates a paternalistic relationship toward the patient, which may undermine consumer organization for mutual self-protection, thereby maintaining consumer atomization. Essentially, it persuades the patient that he need not protect his own interests, either by himself or by organized action. Through atomization of the public into vulnerable patients, paternalism results in the profession's dealing with fragmented individuals instead of bargaining groups. Moreover, by appealing to patient salvation fantasies, trust inducement can stimulate interpatient competition by increasing each patient's desire to see that nothing stand between the doctor and himself. Much of the emotional power of the sentiment of the "doctor-patient relationship" resides in this wish of the patient to save himself at any cost to himself or others. When sick or dying, the patient is most likely to see any obstacle between himself and the doctor as a personal threat. Consequently, the patient becomes willing to accept the profession's desire not to deal with outside parties for the sake of privileged access to services—just in case. Yet another monopolistic consequence is the use of trust inducement to legitimize licensing privileges. Since legislators and other political figures cannot usually judge the quality of medical services, trust inducement plays a major role in political persuasion for obtaining legal privileges.

Consultations among physicians occupy a large part of Percival's work. The basic rule of conduct covering them is worth quoting in its entirety:

> Consultations should be promoted in difficult or protracted cases, as they give rise to confidence, energy and more enlarged views in practice. On such occasions no rivalship or jealousy should be indulged. Candour, probity and all due respect should be exercised towards the physician or surgeon first engaged. And as he may be

presumed to be best acquainted with the patient and
with his family, he should deliver all the medical directions agreed upon, though he may not have precedency
in seniority or rank.[3]

In other words the consulting physician should conduct the
consultation in the presence of the doctor who called him
into the case. Both physicians should try to arrive together,
examine together "that the unnecessary repetition of questions may be avoided," and discuss the case together with
the patient or his friends only after having agreed on what
the patient should be told and what the prognosis should
be. Protracted consultations with a doctor "objectionable
to the patient" should be limited to two or three visits, and
the consulted physician should be given "a double gratuity"
for an "extraordinary portion of both time and attention,"
presumably to compensate him for having to deal with an
unpleasant and unappreciative patient. Consultations should
be preferred with physicians with "a regular academic education," but can be had with an uneducated "intelligent practitioner" for "the good of the Patient."[4]

   These rules for consultations bear one major and one minor
relationship to monopolization. Their manifest purpose, of
course, is to prevent disputes so that doctors will share
information and skill. The rule which maintains the attending physician's control, however, and the admonition against
rivalry appear to be anticompetitive devices. Though encouraging consultation might be interpreted as encouraging group
solidarity, it is probably equally important as a group integrative device for encouraging membership loyalty. Consultations distribute income among group members as well as
information and skill, and such distribution can be important
in times of oversupply of practitioners. And since consultations add another fee to a patient's case, they may bring
a greater total income into the profession. So, anticompeti-
tion is the major purpose of these rules, and group integration
a minor one. The rule permitting consultations with uneducated practitioners is interesting in historical retrospect and

[3] *Ibid.*, p. 38.
[4] *Ibid.*, sections VII, VIII, X-XII, pp. 94-97.

does not seem to contribute to the group's monopolization or institutionalization. It is interesting because of a later movement in the United States to prevent exactly such consultations, a clearer example of monopolistic restrictionism. In this area, at least, Percival's ethics are not as monopolistic as they might have been. The rules discouraging competition, however, are still applicable in any oversupply situation, whether prior to the creation of modern restrictive systems of medical education or currently in certain over-staffed urban areas.

Percival also pays considerable attention to the problem of taking over another physician's patient. A physician called in by a patient on a case not helped by another physician should first consult with the previous physician, ostensibly to better understand the case. If the patient has already contacted the physician, perhaps during a visit with another patient of the physician, the previous physician's general plan of treatment should be followed, unless conditions warrant otherwise, in which case the previous physician should be consulted. An anxious patient who cannot wait for a consultation should be similarly handled. A physician should intervene on his own judgment only if consultation is precluded by "the lateness of the hour" or the urgency of the situation. No consultation is called for when taking over for a sick or absent physician. A physician who is questioned by a patient about treatment by another physician need not consult with the other physician but "should not interfere in the curative plans pursued; and should even recommend a steady adherence to them, if they appear to merit approbation."[5] In short, in such cases, a physician should continue the initiated therapy and, when possible, praise it if he can.

Essentially, these rules discourage criticism and thereby contribute to monopolization. They are in this respect more important for the institutionalization of the profession than are rules of consultation. Like rules of consultation, they discourage competition for patients by preventing patients from comparing the advice of physicians and "shopping around." The noncompetitive, cooperative implications of

[5] *Ibid.*, sections. VI, VIII, XIV, XXVI, XXVII, pp. 93-97.

consultations apply here as well. Self-silencing of criticism prevents the breakdown of patient and public trust in the profession and so plays an additional role in monopolization: inhibiting external controls on the profession. A breakdown of trust can lead to consumer protective organizations, as has been suggested; open criticism can undermine professional claims of keeping its own house clean and invite governmental controls. Insofar as monopolization includes policy-making authority, external controls narrow the range of legitimate professional policy making and thwart monopolization. That controls in one area of professional policy making, such as quality or costs, would lead to controls in others is probably not inevitable, yet one gets the impression that professional leaders see monopolistic powers as interdependently woven upon the same assumption: loss of one privilege might undermine all. So, these rules reduce both internal competition and external controls, protecting the group from dissolution into individualized practitioners.

Percival also offers rules for economic conduct, all of which are variants of the principle of the sliding scale (different fees for patients who meet certain criteria). The basic rule was set in honorific terms:

> Some general rule should be adopted by the faculty in every town relative to the pecuniary acknowledgements of their patients, and it should be deemed a point of honour to adhere to this rule with as much steadiness as varying circumstances will admit. For it is obvious that an average fee, as suited to the general rank of patients, must be an inadequate gratuity from the rich, who often require attendance not absolutely necessary, and yet too large to be expected from that class of citizens who would feel a reluctance, in calling for assistance, without making some decent and satisfactory retribution.[6]

Payment, furthermore, should be based on the economic standing of the patient and not of the physician. Percival

---

[6] *Ibid.*, section XV, pp. 98-100.

specifically warns of the danger in not always charging "the affluent, because it is an injury to his professional breathren. The office of physician can never be supported but as a lucrative one; and it is defrauding, in some degree, the common funds for its support, when fees are dispensed with, which might justly be claimed."[7] Consultations by letter should be charged doubly, because it "imposes much more trouble and attention than a personal visit." While the poor should pay less, some patients should pay nothing. Patients otherwise under the care of a sick or absent physician, mendicant clergymen, military and naval subaltern officers, and "persons who hold situations of honour and trust in the army, the navy, or the civil departments of government" who require sickness certificates all should be treated gratis as "acts due to the public and therefore not to be compensated by any gratuity."[8] Physicians, surgeons, and their immediate families are also to receive free care.[9]

While a sliding scale does not seem to be as monopolistic as uniform fees, there is little question that it is economically rational, at least when there is a shortage of patients. To accept whatever patients can afford is more profitable than to turn away those who cannot afford a fixed fee. At the same time, Percival opposed competing for patients when he opposed undercharging the affluent. He is at first confusing when he claims that wealthy physicians should maintain full fees in behalf of the profession's collective solvency, since the members of the profession do not share income. He implies, however, that a physician may collect all he can from a patient but should not collect less, for price competition might develop. The temptation is particularly great for wealthier physicians who can afford to charge less, perhaps for the sake of prestige, and divert solvent patients from poorer physicians. In this sense, Percival is correct that maintaining full fees helps the profession's collective solvency, but only because wealthier physicians forego a competitive advantage. It also furthers professional solidarity by encouraging physicians to think of their mutual interests.

[7] *Ibid.*, p. 105.
[8] *Ibid.*, p. 102.
[9] *Ibid.*, sections XIV, XV, XVI, XVIII-XX, XXV, pp. 98-103, 105.

The monopolistic effects of the provision of free care to certain groups may not be as clear as for other rules, yet they are present. It could be interpreted as the creation of political allies by morally indebting strategically placed officials and influential persons. Unfortunately, if these people were not in positions where they could help the profession politically, winning a sense of obligation might have been useless. Nonetheless, discounting the cost of care for those with whom solidarity might be useful potentially contributes to monopolization. While a physician's emotional ties might indeed harm his technical judgment when treating his family, free care by an unrelated physician also builds professional solidarity by making treatment a less economic and more personal relationship. It helps the physician feel he is a special person, set off from the rest of society, tied through bonds of generosity and love to other members of the profession. Consequently, this quasi-fraternal device makes the physician more emotionally committed to protecting and furthering the interests of the profession and in general more disposed to accepting the cooperative attitudes which help form the profession into a unitary supply source. Similarly in this spirit of cooperation, doctors are expected to help one another out for a short time by taking over gratis the care of a patient when necessary. These devices are conducive to professional solidarity and help reduce nonmonopolistic competition. More important, however, by accepting responsibility for even the poor, Percival declares a monopoly for physicians over the care of all patients. This claim for authority over the medical market, as I shall later show, is not as economically rational or as effective a method of actual domination of the market as is the setting of fixed fees. But as part of the emergent ideology of the modern medical profession, it seems consistent with attempts to eliminate external competitors.

In other passages, Percival calls on physicians to defend the honor of the profession by withholding criticism:

The *Esprit de Corps* is a principle of action founded in human nature, and when duly regulated, is both rational and laudable. Every man who enters into a fraternity engages, by a tacit compact, not only to submit to the laws, but to promote the honour and interest of the association, so far as they are consistent with morality, and the general good of mankind. A physician, therefore, should cautiously guard against whatever may injure the general respectability of his profession; and should avoid all contumelious representations of the faculty at large; all general charges against their selfishness or improbity; and the indulgence of an affected or jocular skepticism, concerning the efficacy and utility of the healing art.[10]

Physicians should refrain from criticizing individual practitioners as well as the profession as a whole. A physician should not publicly criticize another for incompetence uncovered during a consultation or during treatment of another's patients taken over for a while, or for incompetence discovered in any other way. Other means for influencing the course of treatment should be employed privately. He should also not make public the existence of controversies over the proper course of treatment; he should submit such controversies in private to an arbitration board of professionals, who may then make a public stand.[11]

Percival's comments on criticism fall into two broad categories: criticism of the profession as a whole and criticism of individual practitioners. As will be seen, they overlap in certain respects. Criticism of the profession as a whole is antimonopolistic in the sense that it opposes trust-inducement devices. This association to trust is contained in the functionalist argument as well, that is, that physicians should do nothing to make patients mistrust their physician, for care will be more difficult to perform. The monopolistic consequences of trust inducement, to repeat, are commodity creation, integration of physicians, consumer atomization, and inducement of legal privileges. And to the extent that criticism undermines trust, it also undermines these monopolistic consequences.

[10] *Ibid.*, pp. 104-105.
[11] *Ibid.*, sections IV, IX, XIV, XXIII, XXIV, pp. 92-93, 95-96, 98, 104-105.

Criticism of individual practitioners undermines monopolization through three mechanisms. It can be a competitive device for winning over patients from other physicians, i.e., a market substitute for lower fees. Criticism can invite outsiders to apply self-protective controls on professional activities by implying that the profession cannot regulate itself or "keep its own house clean." Criticism of individual practitioners can also contribute to criticism of the profession as a whole, since failure to self-regulate implies misplacement of public trust in the profession. All criticism is antimonopolistic in another sense: it tends to counter the fraternalization of practitioners, even when made in private. It is a latent source of conflict which can divide the profession and lead to group dissolution. For criticism not to have such effects, it must be set off from normal interaction and defined as impersonal. Percival, however, does not touch on this problem of private criticism. On the basis of this analysis of Percival's work, I can say in summary that criticism in public is antimonopolistic, because it destroys trust, invites countermonopolistic actions by outsiders, and can act as a competitive device.

Percival includes a section on the moral importance of looking back at cases to learn from them:

At the close of every interesting and important case, especially when it had terminated fatally, a physician should trace back, in calm reflection, all the steps which he had taken in the treatment of it. This review of the origin, progress, and conclusion of the malady; of the whole curative plan pursued; and of the particular operation of the several remedies employed, as well as of the doses and periods of time in which they were administered, will furnish the most authentic documents on which individual experience can be formed. But it is in a moral view that the practice is here recommended; and it should be performed with the most scrupulous impartiality. Let no self-deception be permitted in the retrospect; and if errors, either of omission or commission, are discovered, it behooves that they should be

brought fairly and fully to the mental view. Regrets may
follow, but criminality will thus be obviated. For good
intentions, and the imperfections of human skill which
cannot anticipate the knowledge that events alone dis-
close, will sufficiently justify what is past, provided the
failure be made conscientiously subservient to future
wisdom and rectitude in professional conduct.[12]

The retrospection clause is interesting from a monopolization perspective because of its expectations about the
behavior of others. To the extent that it is interpretable as
an injunction against criticism of individual practitioners,
the clause shares the monopolistic consequences of all such
injunctions. Since the retrospection clause excuses poor
practice if the physician learns from his mistakes, however,
it tends to favor leniency and carelessness. The relationship
of this clause to trust-inducement, then, is ambiguous. It
might undermine public trust by announcing that physicians
make mistakes—recognizing human fallibility only reduces
moral responsibility; it does not reassure the patient that
errors will not occur—and by not calling for penalties for
errors. So it might seem antimonopolistic. But allowing in
a semipublic document such as a code of ethics that physicians err is more than compensated for by concealing errors
in everyday practice. And leaving accountability for mistakes
to individual conscience rather than collective professional
action—a notable omission in Percival—amounts to a suppression of both public and private internal criticism.

The 1847 "Code of Ethics" of the American Medical
Association states well the implications of Percival's individualistic statement about retrospection. Care for the sick, it
held, constitutes an obligation "the more deep and enduring,
because there is no tribunal, other than his own conscience
to adjudge penalties for carelessness or neglect."[13] One would
thus expect official actions against incompetence to be low
in the profession. Some evidence bears this out. In America,
incompetence has rarely been grounds for license revocation.

[12] *Ibid.*, pp. 106 ff.
[13] *Ibid.*, p. 219.

In New York State, for instance, 230 complaints of unprofessional conduct and malpractice registered with the State Licensing Board between 1926 and 1939 resulted in only one disciplinary action and no suspension or revocation of license. In 1961, only five states disciplined physicians in any way for professional incompetence.[14]

A study of 938 "disciplinary actions" by state licensing boards between 1963 and 1967 suggested little change. Only seven actions were due to "gross malpractice" (0.7 percent); the type of action (revocation or reprimand) was not specified. These figures may not be complete, no uniform centralized statistical compilation exists, and the author of these recent studies had to compile his figures from the files of the Federation of State Medical Boards of the United States. His 1965 study found that only seven states had laws against both mental and physical incompetence; eighteen had provisions for physical or professional incompetence (defined as the inability to perform medicine), and twenty-seven covered mental incompetence specifically. Twelve states had no specific legal provisions for medical incompetence in any form. Indeed, "The constitutions and bylaws of 38 state medical societies did not specify incompetence as a cause for action against their members. In the states which did have such provisions, members could be expelled for incompetence. But only seven societies had ever disciplined physicians because of incompetence."[15] These observations are consistent with a Percivalean reluctance to have professionals declared incompetent by the profession. Ethics could have exerted force as determinants of the profession's social organization, and so their latent monopolistic implications may well have had practical consequences.

Percival had some miscellaneous passages which bear varying degrees of relevance for monopolization. They are mentioned here only for the sake of thoroughness. Physicians called in to treat another physician's family should offer

[14] Robert Feinbaum, "The Doctor and the Public: A Case Study of Professional Politics" (Doctoral dissertation, Department of Sociology, University of California, Berkeley, 1967), p. 32.

[15] Robert C. Derbyshire, *Medical Licensure and Discipline in the United States* (Baltimore and London: John Hopkins Press, 1969), pp. 77, 79, 87.

sincere advice but leave the final decision to the summoning physician regardless of rank, seniority, or other considerations. His rationale is that "the mind of a husband, a father, or a friend may receive a deep and lasting wound, if the disease terminated fatally, from the adoption of means he could not approve, or the rejection of those he wished to be tried."[16] The consequences for monopolization in this passage are minimal. Quack medicines are not to be used even if the patient wishes them; they would, one might think, be the methods of those outside the interest group and might be interpretable as an endorsement. Another passage calls for the rigid separation of "the provinces of physic and surgery" on the grounds that each has its special area of expertise. Though this sounds paternalistic through assuring competence, it is more precisely an acknowledgment of the status pretensions of the Royal College of Physicians of London, which had asserted its superiority over the surgeons for centuries.[17]

The examination of Percival's *Medical Ethics* has contributed several insights to this study. Using Weber's theory of monopolization, I have specified which of Percival's medical ethics have had monopolistic consequences and the manner in which these ethics have been monopolistic. In at least one instance, the retrospection clause, I have demonstrated how they have probably influenced official professional institutions. Presumably similar demonstrations might be offered for other ethics but will not be here, since such an examination would exceed the limits of this study. I have not, however, discussed to any appreciable degree other possible consequences of medical ethics, for example, for the patient's medical interests or for the distribution of health care. That ethics have multiple consequences seems obvious, but I have selected those components which seem most relevant to the problem of the profession's institutionalization. Nor have I explained the origin of these ethics. The intent behind writing these ethics is simply not well enough documented for me to draw any convincing conclusions. True enough, Weber's

[16] Leake, *op. cit.* (n. 1, above), p. 101.

[17] Joseph F. Kett, *The Formation of the American Medical Profession: The Role of Institutions, 1780-1860* (New Haven and London: Yale University Press, 1968), p. 2.

monopolization model assumes that a concern with maximizing the group's interests drives the process of monopolization, but there is nothing in Percival's *Medical Ethics* consistent or inconsistent with this assumption. All I can say is that to the extent that Weber's assumption is accurate, one can reconstruct Percival's ethics in an unexpected and penetrating way.

My point is that ethics can be a potent organizational tool or resource. They can serve group interests as well as patient medical interests by acting as a tool for ordering conduct in a monopolistic direction. They can help subordinate individual interests to the collective interests of the profession. Many of these ethics require that individual practitioners sacrifice economic or other rewards for the sake of fellow practitioners. They require affluent physicians to forego the prestige of caring gratis for wealthy patients, and prohibit price competition, secret nostrums, self-praise and criticism of others, and a number of other personal rewards, for the sake of the general welfare of the profession as a whole. In the long run, everyone may benefit over and above the returns of individual action, but cooperative action requires some measure of self-sacrifice. Ethics are important in this context, because they provide the means for promoting self-sacrifice and organizing men to pursue their common interests. As appeals to honor, they are "status conventions" (Weber) and answer the Marxian problem of how to transform a class-in-itself into a class-for-itself by using the integrative effects of status interests. Ethics, then, are to be singled out as a very important means for bringing about interest-group cooperation in the medical profession. They are also important as means for discouraging external controls which might interfere with monopolization. Status conventions contribute to monopolization, especially to the extent that they contain latent monopolistic consequences. Thus, they become important organizational tools in an overall monopolization strategy.

Earlier medical ethics

Medical ethics can serve as organizational tools for a monopolization strategy, but they can have other organiza-

tional uses as well. Medical ethics are interesting because
they latently dictate ideal relationships between physicians.
They can suggest, sometimes through inference, how some
physicians thought they could best handle the problem of
interest pursuit, and how they thought each other's interests
were related. I will address several questions along these lines.
If one looks at earlier codes than Percival's, will one find
similar assumptions about how doctors should be and can
be organized? If not, what *are* the social ideals expressed
by those codes, and what social theory assumptions do they
contain? Furthermore, how did these codes answer the problem of interest satisfaction for physicians? Have other medical ethics served as organizational tools in a sense different
from Percival's? Finally, can a comparative study of medical
ethics help clarify the organizational uses of Percivalean
ethics?

Before beginning the comparative study of ethics, one
should try to understand Percival's ethics by itself as a
coherent social theory. I have already discussed its appropriateness as an instrument for a monopolization strategy.
Where does Percival stand, however, with respect to several
issues in social theory?

One of the most conspicuous themes in Percival's medical
ethics is his opposition to any form of competition. He
opposes price competition and any claims which might distinguish one physician from another, i.e., quality competition. This is in marked contrast to the deep interest in
competitive devices of one of Percival's contemporaries, the
liberal Adam Smith. Since Smith's *Wealth of Nations* was
published in 1776, one would expect that an educated man
such as Percival was familiar with the arguments of Smith.
Even though Percival never mentions Smith, he appears to
have responded to liberalism in his code of ethics. Unlike
Smith, Percival also opposes individualizing tendencies in
social organization. Seeing dangers such as unchecked exploitation by individual practitioners, Percival favors the
idea of a principled honorable fraternity of self-denying
practitioners. One of his arguments in behalf of professional
silence, in fact, hits at the dangers of individualized medicine;
he is troubled by Montaigne's complaint about physicians.

"That they perpetually direct variations in each other's prescriptions. 'Whoever saw,' says he, 'one physician approve of the prescription of another, without taking something away, or adding something to it? By which they sufficiently betray their act, and make it manifest to us, that they therein more consider their own reputation, and consequently their profit, than their patient's interest.' "[18]

Unlike Smith, Percival seriously questions the advantages of relying on economic motives for social organization. Instead of trying to arrange material rewards to maximize certain types of behavior—as would a modern social engineer—Percival wants physicians to transcend their personal motives. He believes in the possibility of virtuous men as the outcome of honorific appeals, and he wishes to solve the problem of power by having physicians be virtuous men. Toward this end, he apparently wants to create an internally consistent body of moral advice which an ideally moral man could follow. He finds consistency a difficult task, and he is clearly upset by this, for instance, when he discusses the dilemma between lying and gloomy prognosticating in fatal cases.[19]

Percival's social theory is two-pronged. He wants an intermediate social group between state and the individual with which physicians can identify; he wants an ethical code to integrate and guide members in their conduct. The purpose of the intermediate group is to provide a sense of status honor to buttress the ethical code, but the preservation and protection of the group is also one purpose of the code.

While one can easily see how the code can serve the group's interests, one has more difficulty with the role of the group in maintaining the code. When Percival declines to call for group sanctions, one wonders how he expects to have virtuous men follow the code without coercion or group controls on behavior. Apparently, he believes that virtuous men of spontaneous good conscience can exist without group regulation and without sanctions. This stand is consistent with his rejection of economic motivation for professional action. Percival evidently believes in the fundamental goodness of

[18] Leake, *op. cit.* (n. 1, above), p. 197.
[19] *Ibid.*, pp. 194-195.

human nature and on this basis rejects the need for sanctions. To assert the need for professional criticism and regulation would impugn the good character of physicians. The ethics in this light are presented as a set of wise ideals which require no punishment for violations. All the group can do is provide a body of men with whom one would be proud to associate. Percival evidently believed in the power of revealed reason: physicians have a single most rational way to behave and, once shown the way, will follow. Percival's role is to be the voice of Reason.

As a social philosopher, Percival stands as a naively saintly man: he disdains conflict, bourgeois competitiveness, and group coercion; he envisions conscientious men, professional identification with a higher cause, and the superiority of ethical wisdom over social controls. Percival embraces the idea of a strong profession composed of strong members committed to the goodness of their cause; how this might be accomplished did not, as with many Enlightenment thinkers, seem problematic to him. Presumably the rationality of men once shown the way would be sufficient.

The literature concerning Hippocratic ethics is large, indeed, but most of the questions it addresses are not relevant for the purpose of this chapter. I am interested in the work of Hippocrates only insofar as it has organizational consequences and elucidates Percivalean ethics. One must look to the *Oath, Law, Precepts,* and *Decorum* sections of the Hippocratic collection for a complete version of the general principles of moral conduct and good taste. In their essentials, these principles are that the physician *should* (a) call a consultant if in doubt, (b) be reasonable in fees, and if necessary or possible, forego them entirely, (c) lead a pure and moral life, trying to be, in the highest sense of the word, a philosopher, and (d) respect and honor his teachers; and that the physician *should not* (a) give nor sanction the giving of a poison, (b) cause nor encourage abortion, (c) use his position to debauch a patient nor any member of the patient's household, (d) divulge information about a patient, whether acquired professionally or otherwise, (e) advertise in any manner, nor (f) assume ostentation in dress or manner, nor annoy patients with noise or odors, especially those of wine.[20]

Most major commentators attempt to establish that the Hippocratic ethics are religious. Edelstein, for instance, strongly argues that despite some utilitarian features, the ethics—particularly the Oath—and religious beliefs of the Pythagorean sect of the fourth century B.C. were perfectly and uniquely consistent. Abortion and suicide, for example, were morally opposed only by the Pythagoreans in ancient Greece. Religious or not, these ethics have a strong ascetic theme. The Hippocratic ethics, I believe, attempted to free physicians of all instrumental ends that might interfere with the pursuit of an ascetic, purified medical goal. Physicians should make themselves independently wealthy only so they no longer have to charge fees. They should abstain from sexual relations with patients and those around the patient to prevent sexual desires from distracting them from treatment. They should not advertise, for advertising might lead to economic consciousness and detract both time and thought from purely professional concerns. They should not be ostentatious in dress or manner, for vanity or excessive self-esteem may lead them to subordinate treatment to prestige. Abortion and aiding suicide are themselves the antithesis of the idealized moral goal of the Hippocratic physicians: to cure and to save life.

Characteristically, the Hippocratic code urges the physician to practice medicine with minimum satisfaction of his personal interests. While Percival also calls upon physicians to sacrifice personal interests, he does so for the sake of the social and political interests of the profession as a collectivity. In contrast to Hippocratic ethics, which Ackerknecht has described as "the reform program of an ethically disposed medical minority,"[21] Percivalean ethics attempt to weld physicians together as a group. While Percivalean ethics have many monopolistic consequences for the market, Hippocratic ethics appear to be merely an attempt by a charismatic group of physicians to create a monopoly on virtue. They set fees

---

[20] *Ibid.*, p. 20.
[21] E. H. Acherknecht, "Zur Geschichte der medizinischen Ethik," in *Praxis* 17 (1964), p. 579. Translation mine.

neither high nor beforehand and seek to treat patients free whenever possible. They do not enjoin embarrassing the profession or criticizing other physicians. They do not try to build professional solidarity. They do not directly try to reduce competition; only the prohibition against advertising and the prescription to consult when in doubt touch on the economic aspects of the monopolistic suggestions which run throughout Percival's work.

An example of medieval medical ethics suggests how self-interestedly individualistic medicine could become. The thirteenth-century Royal Court physician, Henri de Mondeville, published a work on medical conduct which supports the personal profit which can be gained through clever image-management. He was, one might point out, considered to be among the best of the profession.

Like Percival, he denounces quarreling before laymen, gives senior physicians the final word in discussions, calls for truth for relatives but only promises of recovery for patients, and recommends a sliding fee scale. Unlike Percival, he recommends a minimum of consultations, refuses to treat the incurable, and cautions close attention to one's own economic interests. "Surgery is superior to medicine, because among other things it is more lucrative. To receive gifts or money, a surgeon dare not fear stench, must be able to cut like an executioner, politely lie, and be clever. Preventive measures should be applied only for counselors, lawyers or advocates, and prepaid patients. The sick above all want to be cured; the surgeon to be paid."[22] Absent in these ethics is the idea of a unified professional group. Mondeville was concerned with how the physician can best protect his own interests and not the interests of other physicians, particularly within the context of a weak political community, where legal guarantees were uncertain. Therefore, he is led to suggest that patients should pay *before* they receive treatment.

The closest tradition to Percival's ethics was no doubt the statutes of the Royal College of Physicians of London (RCP). Indeed, documents with statutes listed as "penal" in 1543 and "ethical" in 1563 include many ideas later found in

[22] *Ibid.*

Percival's work. A consulting physician may not ethically dismiss the attending physician or change treatment without agreement; only the patient had the right to dismiss his attending physician. Physicians are expected to conduct consultations in private, outside the presence of the patient, and are not to criticize one another in public. A 1601 statute prohibits the use of a remedy or treatment kept secret from the College's officers.

Other "ethical" statutes differ from Percival's ethics: consultation with unlicensed persons carries a fine, bargaining for fees except when previously underpaid is prohibited. Information and even the names of medicines are not to be given to the public, ostensibly to prevent misuse. Curiously, violation of these rules resulted only in fines, as determined by a scale. Expulsion from the College could occur only if the offender protested or resisted punishment; this act constituted a breach of oath.[23]

Most RCP statutes were set forth under the leadership of a Dr. Caius, who introduced a large body of ceremonial ornamentations to the College's affairs. These ceremonial additions in language, dress, organizational structure and meetings are suggestive of European secret societies.[24] The ethics of the period would seem consistent with this development, particularly those denying information about medicines, treatment, and the practice of medicine in general, and even about disputes over a specific patient's care. The reluctance to expel members and their easy reentry into the College is also consistent with a body more concerned with preserving its secret knowledge than with eliminating incompetents. The possession of collective secret knowledge is of course consistent with monopolistic action insofar as the knowledge is sought by buyers, that is, as scarcity creation. In this respect, the College differed from secret societies in that secret societies had little or nothing to sell.

When the Enlightenment began in England, the question

[23] Sir George Clark, *A History of the Royal College of Physicians of London*, 2 vols. (Oxford: Clarendon Press for the Royal College of Physicians, 1964, 1966), pp. 96-97, 180-181.

[24] Georg Simmel, "The Secret Society," in *The Sociology of Georg Simmel*, ed. Kurt H. Wolff (London: The Free Press of Glencoe, Collier-Macmillan, 1950), pp. 355-360.

of the rationality of the corporation system, typified by the RCP, arose. One major system of medical ethics, John Gregory's, specifically attacked the monopolistic medical corporations. John Gregory was a professor at the great medical school at Edinburgh, and presumably his independent position there influenced his conclusions about the problem with organized practitioners. His ethics found considerable following. They were written in 1770, circulated widely, found popularity on the Continent during the early nineteenth century, and were promoted in postrevolutionary America by Benjamin Rush.[25]

Gregory's writings on the obligations of the physician to the patient are similar to those Percival later wrote and will not be reviewed here. Unlike Percival, he suggests few regulations for intraprofessional relations, the so-called "medical etiquette," except for consultations even with nonregular physicians and no "arrangements with apothecaries," such as kickbacks and fee splitting.

Gregory's ethical code, however, stands in opposition to the monopolistic codes of the RCP and of the later Percivalean work. Percival saw the forces binding the profession into a group—esprit de corps, a common academic training, and support of each other's reputations—as the source of the best in medicine, as something to be encouraged. Without this group basis, medicine would lose its professionality and hence its excellence. Gregory challenged this central presumption and thereby also the medical profession's elitist autonomy as an independent institutional body. The domination of medical thought by men of the practicing profession, he explained, distorted the pursuit of medical knowledge and blocked the development and delivery of medical care. The profession offered a set of personal ends to physicians other than the furthering of knowledge:

> Much wit has indeed, in all ages, been exerted upon our profession; but after all, we shall find that this ridicule has rather been employed against physicians than physick. There are some reasons for this sufficiently obvious. Physicians, considered as a body of men, who

[25] Ackerknecht, "Zur Geschichte," p. 580.

live by medicine as a profession, have an interest separate and distinct from the honour of the science. In
pursuit of this interest, some have acted with candour,
with honour, with the ingenuous and liberal manners
of gentlemen. Conscious of their own worth, they dis-
dained every artifice, and depended for success on their
real merit. But such men are not the most numerous
in any profession. Some impelled by necessity, some
stimulated by vanity, and others anxious to conceal
ignorance, have had recourse to various means and
unworthy arts to raise their importance among the
ignorant, who are always the most numerous of mankind. Some of these arts have been an affectation of
mystery in all their writings and conversations relating
to their profession; an affectation of knowledge, inscru-
table to all, except the adepts in the science; an air of
perfect confidence in their own skill and abilities; and
a demeanor solemn, contemptuous, and highly expres-
sive of self-sufficiency. These arts, however well they
might succeed with the rest of mankind, could not escape
the censure of the more judicious, nor elude the ridicule
of men of wit and humor. The stage, in particular, has
used freedom with the professors of the salutary art;
but as is evident, that most of the satire is levelled
against the particular notions, or manners of individuals,
and not against the science itself.[26]

He criticizes two characteristics of the profession: formalism
and restriction of knowledge. The formalities which the
profession institutes to appear dignified can interfere with
the primary purposes of the profession as a liberal discipline
devoted to medical science and the care of humanity. Considerations such as the university where a physician obtains
his degree or even the possession of a medical degree are
to be overridden by the plight of the patient:

It is a physician's duty to do everything in his power
that is not criminal, to save the life of his patient, and

[26] John Gregory, *Lectures on the Duties and Qualifications of a Physician*
(London: Strahan and T. Cadell, 1772), p. 60.

to search for remedies from every source, and from every hand, however mean and contemptible. This, it may be said, is sacrificing the dignity and interests of the faculty. But I am not here speaking of the private police of a corporation, or the little arts of a craft. I am treating of the duties of a liberal profession, whose object is the life and health of the human species, a profession to be exercised by gentle men of honour and ingenuous manners; the dignity of which can never be supported by means that are inconsistent with its ultimate objects, and that only tend to increase the pride and fill the pockets of a few individuals.[27]

The attempts by physicians, surgeons, and apothecaries to separate each other's domains, while reasonable to the extent that men should preferably do what they can do best, should be complied with only if the patient's welfare is not sacrificed. In fact, separation into the three domains is prudent and imprudent for the same reason: meritorious skill and liberal knowledge best serve the patient. When the formality of separation comes before the judicious application of skill and knowledge, the patient is wronged:

As a doctor's degree can never confer sense, the title alone can never command regard; neither should the want of it deprive any man of the esteem and deference due to real merit. If a surgeon or apothecary has had the education, and acquired the knowledge of a physician, he is a physician to be respected and treated accordingly. There are certain limits, however, between the two professions, which ought to be attended to; as they are established by the customs of the country, and by the rules of their several societies. But a physician, of a candid and liberal spirit, will never take advantage of what a nominal distinction, and certain privileges, give him over men, who, in point of real merit, are his equals; and will feel no superiority, but what arises from superior learning, superior abilities, and more liberal

[27] *Ibid.*, pp. 39-40.

manners. He will despise those distinctions founded in vanity, self-interest, or caprice; and will be careful, that the interests of science and mankind shall never be hurt by a punctilious adherence to formalities.[28]

Gregory's second criticism struck more directly at the type of professional organization Percival and other conservatives advocated: an autonomous, self-regulating body of elitist experts who made a living by treating patients and who sought to maximize the distance between medical man and patient, using secrecy and systematic ignorance to accentuate the disadvantageous position of the patient. Gregory believed, however, that confining practice "entirely to a class of men who live by it as a profession, is unfavorable to the progress of the art."[29] The love of and devotion to medicine as an art, differentially distributed among physicians, "is often checked by a necessary attention to private interest." In most arts compromise by private interest is acceptable because "all mankind are judges." But in the case of medicine and of medicine alone, the public is in no position to judge the merit of a practitioner; medical practice is too private and medical science kept too secret.[30] A physician with an acquaintance with "the outlines of practice," good presence, and good sense can persuade the public of his merit and become successful, for the public assumes that a physician clever in nonmedical matters will also be good in medicine. Gregory was taken aback, however, by the success of some incompetents who had little to recommend them even outside of medicine. The public could not seem to judge good physicians even by analogy. Like the conservative, then, Gregory concluded that the public could not judge accurately the technical merit of a physician.

Gregory posed for himself this problem: granted, the public cannot evelute physicians accurately and so cannot direct itself to the best doctors; only the physician's own profession can judge his merit and direct patients to men of superior merit; *but* the collective interests of the practicing profession

[28] *Ibid.*, p. 62.
[29] *Ibid.*, p. 213.
[30] *Ibid.*, p. 215.

require that superior merit be concealed so that competition not occur.[31] Therefore, the private interests of the profession led to the concealment of information which might benefit the medical interests of patients.

Gregory also saw other disadvantages to leaving medical knowledge solely in the hands of practitioners. Thorough, careful research can best be done by a man whose practice does not take up his time or distract his attention. Freedom to question existing practices and knowledge is also more available to the gentleman who is not bound to adhere to a systematic body of professionally acceptable procedures and treatments. In fact, the quack has a scientific advantage over the legal practitioner in that he can depart with impunity from conventional methods to experiment with something new, whether a drug or a procedure. The quack does not often contribute to science, however, because his ignorance prevents him from carrying out useful experiments or recognizing important results when they occur.[32]

Gregory's solution was to encourage medical learning outside of the confines of the practicing profession. He thus advocated review of merit by men of liberal education (i.e., gentlemanly education) versed in medicine, who did not practice medicine for a living; they would be least likely to let personal economic interest interfere with a just judgment. Such gentlemen, moreover, would not be hurried by the pressures of their business to provide only a cursory examination and would "possess that tranquility of mind which is so requisite in every kind of investigation."[33] Gregory's comments were directed toward "gentlemen" who were by definition literate and liberally educted; yet they might as well have been applied to anyone with education. Gregory's position was that, for the layman, any knowledge of medicine is better than none. The task, then, was to educate nonpractitioners in medicine, a task he found plausible. "Surely it is not a matter of such difficulty, for a gentleman of a liberal education, to learn so much of medicine as may enable him

[31] *Ibid.*, p. 216.
[32] *Ibid.*, pp. 219-223.
[33] *Ibid.*, pp. 218-220.

to understand the best books on the subject, and to judge
of merit of those physicians to whom he commits the charge
of his own health, and the health of those more immediately
under his care and protection."[34] His criticism of the practicing profession, then, became an analysis of the causes of
public inability to evaluate practitioners. As a consistent
rationalist, he believed that if the public or even some among
the public were sufficiently well educated, competent practitioners would not be placed at a disadvantage.

Knowledge of medicine could be put to many other uses.
In an emergency when a physician cannot be reached, the
knowledge could be helpful. Quacks would not flourish as
widely or cause as much harm if they, as well as the public,
were more knowledgable and less receptive to quasi-magical
remedies. Finally, those who cannot afford medical care
would suffer less harm by drawing more on science and less
on the folklore of nature cures. "Patients are so far from
being left to nature, when no physician is called, that they
are commonly oppressed with a succession of infallible cures
recommended by quacks or their weak and officious
friends."[35] It would, in turn, effect a good influence on the
medical profession to have a well educated public, for physicians would then be conduced to improve their technical
skill rather than develop sales techniques for "the most
ignorant, and consequently the most conceited part of mankind," the public with its prejudices and caprices born of
ignorance.[36]

The division between Percival's conservative and Gregory's
liberal versions of Enlightenment medicine is best captured
in Gregory's concluding comments. For Percival, the Enlightenment and rationality were available only to elites
paternalistically bound to assuming the burden of protecting
the public. For him, the only conceivable authority in medical matters was the practicing medical profession as represented by the licensing bodies of the Royal Colleges. In his
perspective, if physicians would only rise above the tempta-

[34] *Ibid.*, p. 228.
[35] *Ibid.*, p. 233.
[36] *Ibid.*, pp. 234-235.

tions of personal interest, society would be well served. Gregory rejected much of this formulation, claiming that the public was capable of assuming more responsibility for its own medical welfare than Percival would allow, and that the medical practitioner compromised some of the goals of the profession. Put another way, Percival tended to identify the practitioner with the profession, while Gregory restricted practitioners to one limited sphere within the profession. (Practitioners permit much harm by letting private interests intrude in the form of increasing the value of medical services through systematically ensuring that the public remain medically ignorant.) By restricting knowledge to practitioners they could hinder scientific research, thereby subverting the fundamental commitment of the medical profession to the growth of medical knowledge.

For Percival, the strength of the profession lay in the corporate body of practicing professionals whose group identity encouraged the development of a personal ethical commitment to mankind. For Gregory, the strength of the profession lay in the individual mind's capacity to uncover medical knowledge and use it, despite the constraints of professional rituals and formalities, authoritarian orthodoxy, and economic inducements to play to the public's medically irrational and irrelevant demands. Above all, economic advantage from medical knowledge was not to be sought at the expense of humanity; professional organization that monopolized and exploited medical knowledge for economic ends was deplorable, not because it traded medical help for money, but because it impeded the spread and development of medical science.

Gregory was much troubled by the problem of creating an elite for the promotion of medical science in the presence of a dominant elite devoted to preserving its favorable position on the basis of demand for its services. The first elite is generated, in principle, by the ability of individuals to be selected on the basis of their meritorious development and dissemination of information. The second is created by the exclusion of practicing competitors by a professional group's monopolization and concealment of expert information, in the manner of a secret society. Gregory also recognized that these elites were not totally compatible: a well-educated public encourages the development of an elite of technically excellent practitioners, if the public is free to select its practitioners; but for this incompatibility to be minimized, information must be allowed and encouraged to spread to all sectors of society. The prime responsibility of the profession, then, is to produce and disseminate medical knowledge:

> I hope I have advanced no opinions in these lectures
> that tend to lessen the dignity of a profession which
> has always been considered as most honourable and
> important. But, I apprehend, this dignity is not to be
> supported by a narrow, selfish, corporation-spirit; by
> self-importance; a formality in dress and manners, or
> by an affectation of mystery. The true dignity of physic
> is to be maintained by the superior learning and abilities
> of those who profess it, by the liberal manners of gentle-
> men, and by that openness and candour, which disdain
> all artifice, which invite to a free inquiry, and thus boldly
> bid defiance to all that illiberal ridicule and abuse to
> which medicine has been so much and so long exposed.[37]

Unlike Percivalean ethics, Gregory's ethics were anti-monopolistic in the extreme, and they disapproved of arrangements which emphasized the profession's collective interests. According to him, the satisfaction of the personal interests of physicians should be turned to the advantage of the patient by spreading knowledge so that competitive meritorious service can be recognized and rewarded. Organizational devices that satisfy the personal interests of physicians without promoting superior care, using appeals to the honor of the profession and other mutually protective devices, should have no place in ethical medicine.

My short comparative study of medical ethics, particularly the examination of the role of personal versus collective interests in medical practice, has revealed considerable vari-

[37] *Ibid.*, pp. 237-238.

ation. Hippocratic ethics attempted to suppress satisfaction of personal interests but said nothing about promoting the collective interests of physicians. Mondeville, on the contrary, legitimized the pursuit of personal interests as one of the important ends of successful practitioners. Both Percival and the Royal College of Physicians advanced the collective interests of the profession over the personal interests of practitioners, but the Royal College used economic punishments to punish violations, while Percival used prestige rewards to compensate for economic losses in practice. Gregory, on the contrary, attacked the promotion of professional collective interests by adopting a modern liberal faith in the efficacy of competition and in the potential rationality of nonpractitioners. Even when these ethical systems have called for protecting the interests of patients, they have proposed different solutions to the role of the physician's interests in medical practice. In short, the interests of physicians have been more problematic than those of patients, at least on the normative level. The role of physician's interests in the protection of patient interests is equally complex. Percival, of course, sees harmony between the two, when mediated through the collective interests of the profession, while Gregory suggests that perhaps the two are an unstable mixture. In any event, the question of the role of physician interests has historically been answered in a variety of ways and has not been resolved simply by rules to protect patient interests.

It is also clear that medical ethics have played a variety of organizational roles at different times in history. The monopolistic role of Percivalean ethics has already been established. As far as modern scholarship has determined, the Hippocratic writings were probably a religious code which integrated physicians into the membership of the Pythagorean sect, that is, which subordinated medical conduct to the general rules of the religion.

Mondeville's "ethics" read like a guide to upward mobility, giving hardnosed advice about what physicians must do to be successful in a world with few legal guarantees. The ethics of the Royal College of Physicians also served monopolistic ends; for the most part they tried to suppress overt competition among physicians. Percival, however, addressed the problem of building group solidarity in the profession to help bolster appeals for noncompetition. Gregory opposed the monopolistic tendencies of the profession and essentially tried to free academics from the domination of the medical licensing corporations.

In short, the social role of medical ethics has changed throughout history, apparently in a direction which rationalizes economic conduct. The discovery of a monopolistic tendency in Percivalean ethics is probably not fortuitous. The affinity between Percivalean ethics and the corporation system is also probably not fortuitous. As the following chapter will discuss, the conservative Percival wrote his ethics at a time when the elitist medical corporations had come under democratic attack, particularly by economic liberals. As an apology for the corporations, Percival's work was superb; as a means for integrating the profession, it was unsurpassed. As an instrument for solidarity, it was particularly suitable for extending the monopolistic controls of the RCP to the newly professionalized surgeons and apothecaries. Therefore, on the basis of this comparative study, one can say that Percivalean ethics were probably an organizational tool for bolstering the system of licensing corporations through the encouragement of monopolistic traditions for all professionals, an important device for suppressing competition between different types of professionals which might have been exacerbated by the appearance of increasing numbers of professional corporations.

The vicissitudes of the AMA's medical ethics

Percival's ethics spread beyond Great Britain, particularly into the English-speaking countries. When the American Medical Association (AMA) was founded in Philadelphia in 1846, for example, it adopted a code of ethics supposedly based on Percival's medical ethics. Though the AMA's 1847 "Code of Ethics" was allegedly only a cleaning up of linguistic oddities, it substantially changed the meaning of a number

of Percival's suggestions. The codes changed several times
again, in 1903, 1912, 1949, and 1957. These changes raise
several questions. How did these changes alter Percival's
ethics as an organizational tool and what relation did they
bear to monopolization? Why did these codes change, and
can these changes throw any light on the relationship of
the medical profession to American society and society in
general? Finally, what conceptual changes does Weber's
theory of monopolization require in light of these new materials?

The most far-reaching issue is the meaning of medical
service. Medical ethics, including the ethics of the AMA,
have defined service differently. The Hippocratic definition
of service was a purified goal of saving life and curing illness.
What either the patient or the physician personally wanted,
whether abortion or euthanasia, could never constitute service if it were not consistent with either curing or saving;
the personal interests of both physician and patient were
subordinated to an objectified absolute moral goal. The fact
that the ancients had few truly curative therapies did not
matter. The mission of the Hippocratic physicians was healing, not simply palliation. Mondeville similarly accepted as
service only the promise to cure. He refused, for instance,
to take on the incurable as patients; that would constitute
fraud. As he wrote: "Above all, the sick want to be cured."
But for him, the satisfaction of the personal wants of patients
constituted service, anything else not being fair to the patient. Percival broadened this definition and insisted on
treating incurable patients. He believed that palliative care
was as important a duty as cure. But in so doing, he expanded
the range of commodities which the profession had to offer,
a sort of diversification of services within a monopolistic
setting. Broadening services on these terms is in the interests
of the profession, inasmuch as it expands the income base
by charging for more than cures, and indeed dissociates the
right to receive payment from the obligation to cure.

Both the 1903 and 1912 "Principles of Ethics" of the AMA
similarly urged diversification when it opposed fee splitting.
The practice was so widespread that many physicians op-

posed this injunction. Those who favored it, however, offered many arguments: referrals to specialists would be on the basis of the greatest kickback and not the greatest skill, the public might think the professions engaged in behind-the-scene economic practices, and the physician should be morally strong enough to collect for the services he rendered. As one Louisville physician argued in 1899, "Why the specialist is called upon to convert himself into a combined detective and collecting agency for the benefit of the practitioner who has had the patient first, and knows exactly how much service he has rendered, and is backed by the legal and moral right to collect for himself, I am unable to see."[38] In fact, the defenders of fee splitting also claimed that the general practitioners found fee collection for referrals difficult, for a referral often did not seem to be a reputable medical service to the patient, though it might have seemed so to the physician. Within the context of the patient's desire to be cured, diagnosis and referral are only instrumental to cure. Referrals, check-ups, and preventive care all are noncurative services that the medical profession has had to legitimize as salable. The practice of fee splitting, therefore, represented a failure to break from the premodern concept of service as cure and was inconsistent with diversification. Not surprisingly, one of the more important arguments against fee splitting was that practitioners failed to place "a proper evaluation on their services."[39] Fee splitting also represented another instance of the subordination of the self-interests of individual practitioners to collective professional interests. The general practitioner stood to gain more by finding a maximum kickback than by charging a basic fee; without this financial advantage, fee splitting probably would not have been as widely practiced as has been alleged. So the injunction against fee splitting furthered monopolization in two ways: diversification through treatment for its own sake and the subordination of practitioner self-interest.

The ethics of the AMA also commented on the ethical

[38] Donald E. Konold, *A History of American Medical Ethics 1847-1912* (Madison: University of Wisconsin Press, 1962), p. 66.
[39] *Ibid.*

status of fees in general. To repeat, the Hippocratic position
was that fees were at best a necessary evil which the physician should try to do without. The Greeks did not face the
ethical problems inherent in how a physician should best
satisfy his needs. One can imagine that under medieval
conditions, of which Mondeville must be taken as representative, the problem of meeting needs without the benefit
of legally guaranteed force led to the ethical stand of taking
the most possible when the patient was in his psychically
most vulnerable moment. Both ethical codes envisioned the
problem of fee provision as a problem of the individual
physician. Percival's code clearly begins the modern consciousness of the economic interests of the profession as a
collectivity, above and beyond the interests of its individual
members. By 1903, the American organized profession had
taken the stand that doctors are ethically bound to collect
fees. To do otherwise would degrade the purported value
of the profession's services and might encourage competitive
undercutting. The President of the AMA in 1899, Mathews,
expressed this positive attitude toward the virtue of fee
collection:

> The physician who willingly allows his *clientele* to dic-
> tate terms to him, or is willing to make reductions to
> suit and please his patients, is doing his profession an
> irreparable injury, and he should be ashamed to do so.
> It is undignified and brings the profession into disrepute,
> besides being unjust. If your services are not worth what
> you have charged for them, say so and take less, but
> do not underrate your services by reductions which are
> ridiculous from a business standpoint. . . .

> But the most despicable character is the man who starts
> in to undercharge his *competitors* in order to advance
> his number of patients. If you are going to be a "cheap"
> doctor, all right, but to use your brother practitioner's
> rate to enhance yourself by "cutting under" you descend
> to the level of the mountebank.[40]

[40] Joseph McDowell Mathews, *How to Succeed in the Practice of Medicine*
(Louisville: Morton, 1902), pp. 111-112.

An astonishing transformation had occurred over the centuries: what had originally been a necessary evil to be overcome to be fully ethical became a principled practice. Good medicine now required charging an "honest" price. What had been defended by Percival as necessary for the very existence of the profession a century later became ethical in itself. As conditions of relative oversupply of physicians gave way during the twentieth century in America to relative undersupply, this attitude contributed to the rapid increase in the income of the profession. This principled drawing of equal fees without any criteria for the needs of the profession seems to have made a substantial contribution to monopolization.

The most distinctive change in American medical ethics was the adoption of fee fixing instead of the sliding scale. While the 1847 "Code" retained the rule that wealthy physicians should charge for services, it omitted the sliding scale altogether. Percival, it may be recalled, had called for each physician to know the means of his patients: "Some general rule should be adopted by the faculty in every town relative to the pecuniary acknowledgements of their patients," but this general rule should be varied according to circumstances.[41] The AMA simply called for "some general rules" to be established in every town or district, relative to pecuniary acknowledgments from their patients, which should be adhered to as "uniformly" as possible.[42] The sliding scale was replaced by what today would be called the "usual, customary, prevailing rate": a uniform charge for everyone in a local area delimited by the local medical society. The 1903 "Principles" went a step further and suggested that "some general rules" be adopted "relative to the minimum pecuniary acknowledgement from their patients." The new code thus permitted a physician to price his services above the going rate, letting him risk pricing himself out of the medical market. The advantage of this permissive upper limit was that a physician could raise his fees for his established following, i.e., his "practice," and increase his income, even though he might not engage in competitive undercutting.

[41] Leake, *op. cit.* (n. 1, above), section XV.
[42] *Ibid.*, p. 235.

In this way, ethical conduct could help maximize both the
profession's collective interests and the individual practitioner's personal interests. The profession could price services
above competitive market value; the practitioner could try
for an income as high as he might command.

The principles of uniform fee setting (fee fixing) and a
sliding scale (fee discrimination) are two types of economic
conduct which can be found mixed in any concrete situation.
Fee discrimination maximizes income per patient; fee fixing
maximizes income per unit service, that is, within the total
market. Their relative economic rationality varies according
to the state of the market: a sliding scale is most rational
in an oversupply market, where maximizing the number of
patients is a problem; uniform fees are most rational in an
undersupply market, where patients are plentiful, and selecting more affluent patients is a challenge. Their consequences
for the distribution of care differ: a sliding scale tries to
provide care for all patients; uniform fees tend to create two
classes of patients—paying and charity patients. In either
system, however, they may prevent some ill people from
becoming patients. A sliding scale may lead to making care
inaccessible to some, using various noneconomic mechanisms; uniform fees may also make care inaccessible by
denying it to those who do not pay. Both also require a
certain amount of noncompetition; they both assume that
physicians will not undercut each other by embracing price
competition. In short, price competition tends to minimize
what patients must pay for services; a sliding scale maximizes
what they must pay; and uniform fees select only patients
who can pay a set minimum. Thus, both fee discrimination
and fee fixing are consistent with monopolization, though
in different ways, for they both require group cooperation
to prevent price competition from making inroads. Since
concrete situations are by and large only imperfectly monopolistic, price competition, price discrimination, and price
fixing may all be present in any given instance.

Most remarkably, all recommendations for setting fees
were omitted entirely in the 1912 "Principles of Ethics" of

the AMA. Only a section prohibiting fee splitting and defending the right of physicians to charge for referrals appears:

Sec. 3. It is detrimental to the public good and degrading to the profession, and therefore unprofessional, to give or to receive a commission. It is also unprofessional, to divide a fee for medical advice or surgical treatment, unless the patient or his next friend is fully informed as to the terms of the transaction. The patient should be made to realize that a proper fee should be paid the family physician for the service he renders in determining the surgical and medical treatment suited to the condition and in advising concerning those best qualified to render any special service that may be required by the patient.[43]

Though the disappearance of rules for economic conduct (except for fee splitting) might be interpretable as an example of actual demonopolization, the profession's contemporary political setting suggests why these rules were omitted in 1912. Following the passage of the Sherman Act in 1890, antitrust prosecution of the profession became possible. As early as 1898, price fixing had been found by the courts to violate section one of the Sherman Act, inasmuch as it gave offenders "the power to charge unreasonable prices had they chosen to do so." Not until 1927, however, was price fixing illegal per se.[44] Antitrust legislation probably was not very threatening to the medical profession at first because of the infrequency of prosecution. But during Taft's administration, antitrust suits, instituted by Attorney General Wickersham from 1909 to 1913, rapidly increased in number and peaked in 1913, the year following the revised code of ethics of the AMA.[45] Presumably, an official document of the

[43] *Ibid.*, p. 269.

[44] A. D. Neale, *The Antitrust Laws of the United States of America: A Study of Competition Enforced by Law* (Cambridge: At the University Press, 1962), p. 35.

[45] "During the 49 years from 1891 to 1939 it had instituted an average of less than nine cases a year and a maximum of 27 cases a year (in 1913) . . . several of the prosecutions instituted by Attorney General Wickersham (1909-1913) called

profession which called for uniform fees was an open invitation for prosecution at a time when the targets of prosecution
were uncertain but increasing in number. So, this instance
of apparent demonopolization may in fact have had profound
and theoretically interesting monopolistic consequences.
This theoretical issue will be addressed again later in this
chapter.

The 1949 "Code of Ethics" also omitted references to
setting fees, but they reappear in the 1957 "Code." By 1957,
the physician's fee was supposed to be "commensurate with
the services rendered and the patient's ability to pay.[46] This
passage apparently tries to combine uniform fees with a
sliding scale, without making clear that these are separate
and somewhat contradictory philosophical positions. At best
this passage represents a return to Percivalean fee discrimination. Why the issue of the patient's ability to pay reentered
medical ethics in America at this late date also seems to
require an explanation in terms of the profession's political
setting, for nothing in the profession's internal organizational
needs for structuring economic conduct accounts for the
swing away from uniform fees. The question of which political developments were crucial will be addressed later.

The ethics of the AMA departed from Percivalean ethics
on a number of other issues as well. Some of these changes
were only marginally significant. American medical ethics, for
instance, added one qualification after another to the ancient
commandment of professional secrecy: the physician was at
first required to divulge information when "imperatively
required to do so" (1847), then when "imperatively required
by the laws of the state" (1903), and then to prevent spread
of a communicable disease (1912). Other changes were not
as marginal. Percival had handled the question of public
awareness of medical controversies by requiring that disputes
be submitted to a professional board of arbitrators for a
public stand. The 1847 ethics of the AMA demanded that

---

for the dissolution of trusts." Fritz Machlup, *The Political Economy of Monopoly:
Business, Labor, and Government Policies* (Baltimore: Johns Hopkins Press, 1952),
p. 184, n. 4.
    [46] "Principles of Medical Ethics" (American Medical Association, 1957), pp.
VI-VIII.

"neither the subject matter of such differences nor the adjudication of the arbitrators should be made public, as publicity in a case of this nature may be personally injurious to the individuals concerned, and can hardly fail to bring discredit on the faculty.[47] This position is even more monopolistic than Percival's, in that it denies the public substantial knowledge of the existence of controversies and so reduces the probability of public criticism and consumer organization.

American medical ethics depart from Percivalean ethics in two other very important areas: permissible consultations and permissible settings for practice.

Percival had said that consultations with intelligent practitioners without academic training were permissible. Presumably such consultations worked both ways: the ethical physician might both send and receive referrals from marginal practitioners. The 1847 "Code of Ethics," however, prohibited consultations with anyone "whose practice is based on an exclusive dogma."[48] This blanket prohibition against all consultations with "irregular" practitioners was modified in 1903 to prohibit only referrals to irregulars. Many physicians had argued that closing off part of the medical market by denying eligibility for care to patients under the care of nonorthodox physicians made little sense. If nonorthodox physicians were going to recruit patients for orthodox physicians, the orthodox physicians could take advantage of this recruitment while simultaneously justifying it as the patient's finally receiving "proper" care. This position stood until 1949, when the "Principles of Ethics" forbade consultations with "cultists": "Such consultation lowers the honor and dignity of the profession in the same degree in which it elevates the honor and dignity of those who are irregular in training and practice."[49] Apparently, by 1949 the AMA had returned to a position similar to that of 1847. The 1957 "Ethics," for reasons to be discussed later, excluded mention of consultations with nonorthodox physicians. So, while

---

[47] Leake, *op. cit.* (n. 1, above), p. 235.
[48] *Ibid.*, p. 229.
[49] "Principles of Medical Ethics," *J.A.M.A.* 140 (25 June 1949), p. 701.

Percivalean ethics had concentrated on eliminating internal competition among licensed physicians, American medical ethics also tried to eliminate external competition by controlling practitioner conduct. As will be argued later, ethical controls were a relatively ineffective means for doing so.

American medical ethics faced up to a different internal competition problem than did Percival and so added a new ethical concern to those of traditional Percivalean ethics. The 1903 "Principles" was the first to confront the problem: "Poverty, mutual professional obligations, and certain . . . public duties . . . should always be recognized as presenting valid claims for gratuitous services; but neither institutions endowed by the public or the rich, or by societies for mutual benefit, for life insurance, or for analogous purposes, nor any profession or occupation, can be admitted to possess such privilege."[50] This prohibition attacked what later was called "contract practice," in which doctors were salaried to provide unlimited services to all members of a voluntary organization. The conventional objection to contract practice was that doctors were made to carry too many patients for the performance of good medicine and that payments for treatment out of the doctor's own pocket tended to impoverish physicians. By demanding fees for services within these institutional arrangements, medical ethics could prevent such abuses of physicians and possibly of patient interests. The AMA disapproved of agencies offering medical services to patients and tried to establish the principle that only the medical profession may set the value of services. Institutional contract practice threatened the monopolistic interests of the profession in a number of ways: it created competition with independent physicians by offering medical services to patients at a low yearly membership charge; undermined the idea that medical services are discrete commodities that possess exchange value; provided patients with an organizational base for potentially opposing the medical profession; and placed in nonprofessional hands the right to make a number of policies about the number of patients doctors would see, the amount of services to be provided, the doctor's

[50] Leake, *op. cit.* (n. 1, above), p. 253.

choice of patients, and other conditions of work. Not all contract practice plans contained these features, but as a type, they presented these threats. Later, the 1912 "Principles of Ethics" specifically attacked contract practice under Section 2: "It is unprofessional for a physician to dispose of his services under conditions that make it impossible to render adequate services to his patient or which interfere with reasonable competition among the physicians of a community. To do this is detrimental to the public and to the individual physician, and lowers the dignity of the profession."[51] This passage is interesting, for it ironically opposes one form of internal competition (between employed and independent practitioners) by appealing to the value of competition among independents, so that a patently non-monopolistic structural feature—competition—acquires monopolistic consequences.

Between 1912 and 1949, the date of the next major ethical revision, the medical profession confronted the growth of a variety of institutions and arrangements that have come to be known as "third parties." Any intervening person or institution between the physician and the patient has usually been called a "third party," but governmental medical plans have usually been carefully separated from so-called "voluntary" medical institutions by the AMA. In the thirty-seven year period, the AMA had to come to terms with a variety of medical institutions that challenged the traditional means of monopolistic control: commercial health insurance plans, specialty clinics such as the Mayo Clinic, prepaid plans such as Kaiser-Permanente, and the Blue Cross and Blue Shield Plans (which were semi-autonomous). Some of these organizations grew with the support of the AMA, some were able to survive by coming to terms with local medical societies, and others had to bring suit against the AMA and its constituent societies.[52] Though the interests of the profession would have favored continued atomization of consumers and equal competition among professionals, these intermediate

[51] *Ibid.*, pp. 268-269.
[52] Herman Miles Somers and Anne Ramsay Somers, *Doctors, Patients, and Health Insurance: The Organization and Financing of Medical Care* (Washington, D.C.: The Brookings Institution, 1961), pp. 292, 347-354.

institutions became established and stimulated the AMA to create criteria to distinguish which third parties would henceforth be unacceptable.

The 1949 "Principles" contains four sections which introduce these criteria. First, institutions "should meet such costs as are covered by the contract under which the service is rendered," i.e., physicians should not have to pay out of their own pockets for services to subscribers.[53] Second, contract practice, defined as "an agreement between a physician or a group of physicians, as principals or agents, and a corporation, organization, political subdivision or individual, whereby partial or full medical services are provided for a group or class of individuals on the basis of a fee schedule, or for a salary or for a fixed rate per capita" was no longer unethical per se if it did not violate the ethical provisions of the "Principles of Medical Ethics" or cause "deterioration of the quality of the medical services rendered."[54] Third, restriction of choice of physician was not unethical per se in the event that a third party "by law or volition . . . assumes legal responsibility and provides for the cost of medical care and indemnity for occupational disability." This section apparently permitted the ethical operation of the health services of the Veterans Administration, a form of restricted choice of physician and the only health service in the United States that could have assumed the broad liabilities demanded by the 1949 "Principles." Fourth, "A physician should not dispose of his professional attainments or services to any hospital, lay body, organization, group or individual, by whatever name called, or however organized, under terms or conditions which permit exploitation of the services of the physician for the financial profit of the agency concerned."[55] But apparently commercial health insurance companies, profit-making organizations, were not considered exploiters of the services of the physician. This clause evidently served as a basis for the AMA to oppose organizational arrangements it did not favor, without making explicit its criteria for exploitation.

[53] "Principles," (1949), op. cit., p. 703.
[54] Ibid.
[55] Ibid.

The criteria that the AMA enunciated should be restated: remuneration for all physician services and costs, maintenance of the quality of services, maintenance of ethical standards, free choice of physician except in the case of broad custodial institutional care, no "exploitation" of services for the profit of others. Aside from asserting the profession's commitment to quality service, the provisions created conditions for a one-way flow of resources into the profession by covering costs incurred in the course of delivering services and by forbidding "exploitation" by others for profit: if anyone should gain profits from medical services, it should be physicians. The Principles also discouraged competition between private and institution-based physicians by calling for free choice of physicians so that patients would not be drawn to low-cost or free sources of care. "Free choice" in this context meant that all physicians should be able to be reimbursed by third parties, regardless of patient preference.

The 1949 criteria were also no doubt a reaction to the European and British health organization experiences. General practitioners under the National Health Insurance system of 1911 and the National Health Service of 1948 in Britain had elected to receive capitation fees, which provided a fixed payment by the government for each patient treated during the year and registered on a doctor's "panel." Whatever costs the physician incurred by treating his panel had to be paid out of the capitation money. Also, since the National Health Service provided free medical services for patients who belonged to the NHS, the market for private practice, while not eliminated, was greatly reduced. Doctors did not have to join the NHS; patients did not have to go to NHS doctors. Yet free choice, as defined by the AMA, was not a feature of the NHS, since the program did not pay for services to an NHS patient delivered by nonparticipant physicians. In Britain this distinction presented no problems, since reportedly nearly 100 percent of general practitioners were enrolled in the NHS.[56] The effect on the private medical market, however, was crushing in Britain,

[56] Rosemary Stevens, *Medical Practice in Modern England: The Impact of Specialization and State Medicine* (New Haven and London: Yale University Press, 1966), p. 183.

and the AMA's ethical opposition to arrangements that might have had similar effects in the United States is very understandable.

The *Journal of the American Medical Association* printed a remarkable speech that suggests the AMA's uneasiness about contemporary events in Britain. This speech, by Clem Whitaker of the public relations firm of Whitaker and Baxter, was the AMA's "Report of the Coordinating Committee," and appeared only three pages before the 1949 "Principles of Ethics." Its relevant part calls on American physicians to oppose developments at home similar to those in Britain for the sake of both patients and the moral fiber of America:

Britain began with compulsory health insurance on a supposedly moderate scale back in 1911. Since then the cancer of socialization has spread to almost every part of the British economy. It has eaten up the Bank of England, the cable and wireless services, civil aviation, the transportation industry, the coal industry, the electric industry and more recently the gas industry, and now it is about to spread to the steel industry.

There were those in Britain, when compulsory health insurance was first proposed, who thought it was a harmless experiment. And some of their cousins live here in America. But today Britain is plunging headlong toward a regimented society that will blot out every vestige of liberty for the British people, unless the tide is turned back.

This truth we know—and this truth we must some way make all America know: when medicine is socialized, the beginning of the end is in sight. It is one of the final, irrevocable steps toward complete state socialism. And at the end of that road is loss of everything that means most to free men.

This, without doubt, is the greatest emergency any of you ever has confronted in all your years of practice. Not just one life hangs in the balance, but the life of a nation is in your hands—a nation that has become the last hope of all the liberty-loving people in the world.

In all reverence, I want to say: Thank God that this House of Delegates and the American Medical Association have accepted the challenge. Thank God for the courage, the sound convictions and tireless energy of American doctors.

This isn't just a heavy obligation that has been laid upon you, and I am sure that you don't look at it that way. This is the greatest opportunity any of us ever will have to serve America, to champion our good way of life and to play a vital part in shaping the destiny of our country. The plague of socialization, with all its demoralizing consequences, has become epidemic throughout most of the world. It has impaired and crippled the productive capacity of great nations and stripped them of their political independence. It has undermined the character, the moral fiber and the individual initiative of untold millions who were once prideful, self-reliant, self-supporting people. It has made them serfs of their own governments, dependent on government for their very existence.[57]

Invoking such important values, Whitaker and Baxter called on the American medical profession to produce a highly mobilized response against a series of governmental plans, starting at that time with Truman's National Health Insurance plan. The preservation of a private medical market was transformed from a parochial medical problem to the level of a great international cause. In comparison, changes in medical ethics, while consistent with this reaction, were a mild response to the problem.

In a number of ways, American medical ethics favored monopolization more than Percivalean ethics did. The expanded concept of medical service which prohibited fee splitting, the call for uniform fees, the increased use of secrecy to maintain public trust, the attack on external competitors, and the attack on internal competition by physicians in organized practices were all more monopolistic than Percival's simple plea for noncompetition and solidarity. Since

[57] "Report of Coordinating Committee," *J.A.M.A.* 140 (25 June 1949), p. 697.

the American medical ethics were written by the AMA rather than by any single person, they should be related to the role of the AMA in monopolization. One issue is the degree to which the AMA could claim control over the conduct of individual practitioners. The 1847 "Code" did not specifically require membership in the AMA for ethical standing but suggested a number of criteria for determining the boundaries of the legitimate profession: a regular medical education, nonadherence to an exclusive dogma, a license to practice from some medical board of known and acknowledged respectability recognized by the association, and "good moral and professional standing in the place in which he resides."[58] As such, the Association claimed the right to decide which practitioners were ethical. The 1903 "Principles," however, called on physicians to join "the organized body of the profession as represented in the community in which he resides." All of these county medical societies should affiliate with state medical societies, and those with the American Medical Association.[59] Even though the AMA had changed the title of ethics from a Code to Principles, and called the document only suggestive and advisory, the implication was still present: an ethical physician must belong to the American Medical Association and its constituent bodies. Those who did not belong could not be ethical physicians.

The 1903 "Principles," however, did not do away with all sanctions. There remained, of course, informal prestige sanctions; but even more important, since the advisory status of the ethics applied only to the AMA, state and local medical societies could still apply a variety of penalties for violations of the AMA's ethics. So, in effect, the AMA claimed the right to determine the conduct of physicians through enforced membership and control at a local level. The 1912 "Principles," however, do not mention any ethical responsibility on the part of physicians to join the AMA and local medical societies. This omission may well have been consistent with the political realities of impending antitrust prosecution. If the AMA had achieved virtually 100 percent

[58] Leake, *op. cit.* (n. 1, above), pp. 228-229.
[59] *Ibid.*, pp. 243-244.

control of the medical profession, it might have become subject to antitrust prosecution as a corporate organization which had eliminated competitors. By permitting physicians ethical status without joining the AMA, the AMA could avoid prosecution by dissociating the corporate entity of the Association from the body of licensed practitioners and by denying Association control of practitioners. The AMA has in fact taken the tack that physicians are independent men whose activities cannot be dictated by medical societies; medical societies cannot command where to work or what fees to charge. The medical societies can still declare specific activities unethical and refuse or terminate membership in the society, but constraining limits are not authoritative commands issued by the AMA. This absence of demonstrable organizational authority over the behavior of physicians, in the sense of issuing commands, may have helped prevent antitrust prosecution of the AMA and in any event helps explain why the role of the AMA, as spelled out in ethics, changed between 1903 and 1912.

The role of the AMA as an instrument for the cultivation of fellowship, for the exchange of professional experience, for the advancement of medical knowledge, for the maintenance of ethical standards, and for the promotion in general of the interests of the profession and the welfare of the public, in 1903 was later reduced to a "preferable" board of arbitrators to settle differences of opinion between disputing physicians.[60] In contrast to the 1903 document, the 1912 "Principles" provided the AMA with a comparatively passive manifest political role within the profession. By 1949, medical ethics again called for membership in the Association and prohibited association with marginal practitioners. This resurgence of manifest control probably reflects the profession's greater experience with the politics of antitrust prosecution and the discovery that certain types of control are more vulnerable than others.

The preceding examination of American medical ethics has raised certain theoretical problems. On a number of issues, certain codes have been more monopolistic than Percival's, while others at least at first seem less so. Even though

[60] *Ibid.*, pp. 243, 268.

interpreting the call for uniform fees as monopolistic is straightforward, interpreting the removal of ethical regulations for setting fees is ambiguous. One might well say that the retraction of such passages represents actual demonopolization, that these ethics do not order the conduct of physicians in a monopolistic direction. Before so concluding, however, one should realize that a monopolization strategy has multiple components and that manifest demonopolization of this kind may constitute latent monopolization by solving certain requirements for monopolization.

To be sure, as one finds time and again, codes of ethics may contain nonmonopolistic or even antimonopolistic rules; therefore, I have not been trying to demonstrate that everything in the world of medical ethics is monopolistic. My study of ethics so far has attempted to elucidate the ways in which ethics can contribute to the capacity of a group to engage in monopolistic action. In other words, I have so far considered the requirements of economic monopolization, i.e., the organizational requirements for domination of the market, but I have paid insufficient attention to the problem of politically oriented monopolization: the exigencies imposed by constraints from the political community. What are now required are heuristic concepts for the analysis of the political aspects of monopolization. Two such concepts are offered for consideration: the constraints of audiences on ethics, and the divergence of public and private codes of ethics.

One approach to the profession's political setting is the investigation of audiences addressed by the code of ethics. Percival's ethics for the most part addressed only physicians and responded to the political setting simply by encouraging paternalistic attitudes and by currying favor with politically strategic people. The 1847 "Code" specifically addressed both physician and patient, even including long passages about the duties and obligations of the patient to his physician. These were dropped in 1903 because of their adverse effect on public opinion. One prominent theme in them, however, was that patients should be totally loyal to the physician or find another doctor, an alternative to consumer organization for dissatisfied patients.

By 1903, apparently, state legislatures were an important

audience. The fight for state licensing privileges had just been won in the few preceding decades, and the ethics tended to be concerned with justifying these newly won privileges. The compromising of professional secrecy by legal responsibility for testimony on the medical condition of patients, and the replacing of an attack on practitioners of exclusive dogma with a defense of Association practitioners as scientific, tended to affirm the profession's sense of civic duty and reaffirm the scientific basis of licensing restrictions. As I have suggested, by 1912 the United States Justice Department may well have been an audience. Noteworthy in this context is the appearance of the ideology that the profession exists to serve the public good—its "ideal of service to humanity"—an ideology absent in ethical systems prior to 1912. Apparently, appeals to science were insufficient for legitimizing licensing and other monopolistic privileges, and so appeals to public and human service were added. By 1949 the key new audience was probably federal legislators. A whole series of plans for nationalizing health care delivery were countered with a series of principles about what would constitute unethical practice for physicians. Presumably, the message to this audience was that laws should not be made which would violate professional ethics and which would incidentally put the independent practitioner at a competitive disadvantage.

The 1957 "Principles of Ethics," which has so far received minimal attention in this chapter, appears to be an ingenious solution to the problem of conflicting requirements for a monopolization strategy. While the previous AMA codes all bear a common resemblance, this code is much more general and idealistic. It is also much briefer, sufficiently so that it will be reprinted here in its entirety to give a feel for the code and to make known the most current version of the "Principles."

PREAMBLE

These principles are intended to aid physicians individually and collectively in maintaining a high level of ethical conduct. They are not laws but standards by which a physician may determine the propriety of his conduct in his relationship with patients, with colleagues, with members of allied profession, and with the public.

SECTION 1

The principal objective of the medical profession is to render service to humanity with full respect for the dignity of man. Physicians should merit the confidence of patients entrusted to their care, rendering to each a full measure of service and devotion.

SECTION 2

Physicians should strive continually to improve medical knowledge and skill, and should make available to their patients and colleagues the benefits of their professional attainments.

SECTION 3

A physician should practice a method of healing founded on a scientific basis; and he should not voluntarily associate professionally with anyone who violates this principle.

SECTION 4

The medical profession should safeguard the public and itself against physicians deficient in moral character or professional competence. Physicians should observe all laws, uphold the dignity and honor of the profession and accept its self-imposed disciplines. They should expose, without hesitation, illegal or unethical conduct of fellow members of the profession.

SECTION 5

A physician may choose whom he will serve. In an emergency, however, he should render service to the best of his ability. Having undertaken the care of a patient, he may not neglect him; and unless he has been discharged he may discontinue his service only after giving adequate notice. He should not solicit patients.

SECTION 6

A physician should not dispose of his services under terms or conditions which tend to interfere with or impair the free and complete exercise of his medical judgment and skill or tend to cause a deterioration of the quality of medical care.

SECTION 7

In the practice of medicine a physician should limit the source of his professional income to medical services actually rendered by him, or under his supervision, to his patients. His fee should be commensurate with the services rendered and his patient's ability to pay. He should neither pay nor receive a commission for referral of patients. Drugs, remedies or appliances may be dispensed or supplied by the physician provided it is in the best interests of the patient.

SECTION 8

A physician should seek consultation upon request; in doubtful or difficult cases; or whenever it appears that the quality of medical service may be enhanced thereby.

SECTION 9

A physician may not reveal the confidences entrusted to him in the course of medical attendance, or the deficiencies he may observe in the character of patients, unless he is required to do so by law or unless it becomes necessary in order to protect the welfare of the individual or of the community.

SECTION 10

The honored ideals of the medical profession imply that the responsibilities of the physician extend not only to the individual, but also to society where these responsibilities deserve his interest and participation in activities which have the purpose of improving both the health and the well-being of the individual and the community.[61]

The 1957 "Principles" eliminated virtually all regulations concerning consultations, the duty to affiliate with medical societies, restrictions on institutional arrangements, and any stated role of the AMA in medical affairs. Also important are the inclusion of conflicting demands for fees and services as if they were not contradictory: fees "commensurate with the services rendered" are presumably set according to some standard for the evaluation of services; fees set in accordance with "the patient's ability to pay" work against such standardization. Also, the service ideal of "improving both the health and the well-being of the individual and the community" admits that service to individuals may not constitute community service, but does not go very far toward reconciling the two. These ambiguities suggest that the 1957 "Principles" attempts to resolve internal differences by including everything in a sufficiently vague manner as to offend no one yet provide everyone with a sense of ethical conduct. Whatever the political and social functions of the 1957 "Principles," it is no longer a detailed code of regulations for professional behavior but a statement of professional ideals: service to humanity, medical skill, science, moral and legal correctness, free exercise of skills, fair fees, use of consultations, secrecy under most conditions, and responsibility to both individuals and the community. In one sense, no physician can live up to these ethical standards because they are so abstract and general that they result in practical conflicts. In another sense, all physicians could meet these standards because they are stated as ideals, and ideals are understood to be compromised by reality. Infractions cannot reasonably be punished in most cases because physicians can meet these ideals at least to some degree most of the time.

[61] "Principles," (1957), *op. cit.* (n. 46, above), pp. VI, VII.

Vagueness does not, however, imply decline in control. The telling thing about the 1957 "Principles" is that they do not replace the 1949 "Principles of Medical Ethics;" both are in effect. One might argue that the 1957 ethics are but an abstraction of general principles from the 1949 work, but they seem to be quite different documents. The interpretation I offer is that the 1957 ethics and the 1949 ethics address different audiences. Presumably the 1957 ethics are a statement of ideals for public consumption, and the 1949 ethics are detailed private norms for conduct, for which members of the AMA can still be held accountable. By this means, the monopolistic consequences of medical ethics have been made even less public than before.

The comparative study of medical ethics in America has demonstrated that the codes have indeed departed in certain respects from Percival's ethics, at times becoming more monopolistic but at other times losing certain key monopolistic features. I have attempted to maintain the view that medical ethics are an organizational tool for monopolization but have expanded this perspective to see ethics serving this end in different ways. There has probably been a shift in purpose for medical ethics from a Percivalean means for ordering the conduct of physicians to a means for legitimizing the monopolistic privileges of the profession to the powers-that-be and to the public, though this shift has by no means been total. Medical ethics have probably been strained in recent years to serve both functions, and the device of dual codes of ethics—public and private codes—may help ease this strain. The trend toward making monopolistic features of the profession less public suggests that American society may have become in certain respects less receptive to monopolization by social groups, and that relative submersion of monopolistic features of the profession's organization has been the general strategy for dealing with this change in receptivity. This theme will be examined later in the chapter on American licensure.

It is also clear from this study that Weber's theory of monopolization requires more development on the side of the problem of social receptivity to monopolization. Ordering the conduct of the members of interest groups in a monopolistic direction is not sufficient to account for successful monopolization; the interest group must deal as well with the reactions of other social groups and the constraints of institutions and find favorable groundsoil for growth. Thus, monopolization requires not only developing effective organizing tools but also developing mechanisms for dealing with the shifting receptivity of society to the interest group's efforts. A group may try to organize its members in a monopolistic direction, but the group must still eliminate external competitors, win allies, and disarm critics if it is to monopolize successfully.

The limits of medical ethics for monopolization

While medical ethics may serve well as status conventions for organizing physicians for monopolization, and as idealistic statements for reducing political resistance to the profession, they apparently have not been very effective at eliminating external competitors. This was not always clear. At times in American medical history, the profession has been divided over the relative efficacy of ethics and licensure for eliminating external competition. The great debate between the American Medical Association and the New York State Medical Society in 1882 and 1883 illustrates this problem and helps remind us that social actors are not always sure of the most effective strategy to follow.

Two of the AMA's 1847 regulations broke with local organizational traditions: the prohibition of consultations with nonregular physicians and the call for local price fixing of fees. The ethical code of the State Medical Society of New York, incorporated in 1806, had called for precisely the opposite. The medical society was not authorized to infringe on the activities of any legally accredited physician, for the only differences alleged among physicians were intellectual and personal and the public was to be "the natural judges" of these.[62] Since fixing professional charges was believed undignified for the profession, any society member found

[62] Alfred C. Post, et al., *An Ethical Symposium* (New York: G. P. Putnam's Sons, 1883), p. 179.

"guilty of promoting, favoring, or encouraging the members of any medical society in their corporate capacity to form, support, and fix medical charges" would be expelled forever from the society.[63]

When the AMA's crackdown on homeopathists peaked in 1882, the New York State Society bolted from the AMA in protest and called into question the AMA's use of ethical controls. First, the two ethical controls that prohibited consultations with adherents of an exclusive dogma and called for price fixing were declared to be opposed to the true spirit of professionalism. In a symposium published by professional opponents of the AMA's position in 1883, H.R. Hopkins interpreted the contemporary scene, questioning what was actually happening in the name of ethical professionalism:

> The writer cannot find in the rationale of these two clauses of the code of 1849 (the year of ratification by the New York Society), that intelligent discrimination and high professional purpose which characterized the code of our earlier times.

> Neither is there evidence of the existence of that reciprocal relation and confidence which was the prominent feature of the early professional status. But in both clauses, and from both points of view, there is the most unmistakable tendency to develop trade instincts and trade provisions. As an instance of trade policy, there was method in refusing to recognize physicians, who held unapproved doctrines and were candidates for the patronage we had monopolized. As a stroke of commercial policy, this act was materially strengthened by revolutionizing the relations of the profession concerning fees, by the fixing of fee-bills, and by the placing of a trade value upon every possible professional act or service.

> It is a most remarkable instance of consistent sociological development that the sale of licenses to practice a learned profession, the formation of offensive and defen-

[63] H. R. Hopkins in *ibid.*, p. 181.

sive guilds, and the imposition of a money value upon each professional act, should follow each other in close rapid sequence.[64]

Second, the consequences of professional ethics were questioned. The use of a code was challenged on four counts: (1) it led to a "pharisaical spirit" that replaced concern for the spirit of the code with concern for locating loopholes in the letter of the code and encouraged a pretentious "holier than thou" attitude among physicians;[65] (2) it fostered "a spirit of censoriousness in the profession," turning physicians into spies on one another and creating a "star-chamber tradition" within the organized profession; (3) it was selectively applied, ignoring most provisions and usually enforcing only the doctrine of exclusion. Indirectly, it even led to the growth of public sympathy for and support of homeopathy, which was seen as an underdog sect persecuted by the AMA; (4) it was not applied equally as a means of professional self-regulation, for it was violated without punishment by prominent members of the AMA:

> It has often appeared that its provisions could be observed or disregarded at will by men who were prominent and influential, while the obscure and weak alone were expected to implicitly comply with it. Men who have been notorious for their infractions both of its spirit and letter have repeatedly received the honors of the association which created and maintained it; and in every city there are many who violate it without any attempt being made to subject them to discipline.[66]

Third, the right of the AMA to impose a code of ethics on free professionals was challenged. The opponents asserted that the AMA had no authority over the medical profession as a whole and no more authority over its members than its members voluntarily allowed through their local medical societies.

[64] *Ibid.*, pp. 184-185.
[65] S. O. Vanderpoel and L. S. Pilcher in *ibid.*, pp. 37, 52.
[66] L. S. Pilcher in *ibid.*, pp. 38-39.

To those who are conversant with the loose manner these delegateships are tendered—dependent solely upon whether the person selected desires the recreation of the trip—they carry but little weight or importance with the home organizations, and in no manner represent the professional or intellectual force of the locality. They possess absolutely no delegated authority to do any act or thing which shall affect the status or relations of the home societies toward each other or their individual members. It is, then, but sheer presumption for a body, so variably and loosely organized, to dictate to the whole profession of this country an ethical code which smothers individuality and makes the physician but portion of a conglomerate trades-union.[67]

Patently, the argument of the opposition was riddled through with inconsistencies and illogic. To be sure, the opposition rejected the authority of the AMA over individual members but at the same time tried to change the position of the AMA, as though the AMA's authority were valid. It seems that the opposition wanted both an improved ethic and no ethic at all. The New York State Society eventually decided to split ranks from the AMA rather than merely ignore the AMA's censure.

On one theme, however, the opposition remained consistent: the growing tendency of the AMA to develop trades-union characteristics and to apply the ethical code toward that end. The exact nature of the criticism, however, requires specification. Ironically, the AMA had been called into being by the New York State Medical Society at a convention at New York University thirty-seven years earlier in 1846. The intention of the society had been to upgrade the technical quality of regular practitioners in order to defend itself against the accusations of incompetence by "irregulars," particularly by the relatively well educated homeopathists. One New York platform was the institutionalization within each state of legal licensure separate from a diploma.[68]

[67] S. O. Vanderpoel in *ibid.*, pp. 38-39.
[68] Kett, *op. cit.* (n. 17, above), pp. 170-171.

Pressure from medical schools, threatened by the prospect
of instituting well qualified educational programs and of
losing income from students unwilling to attend long periods
of formal lectures, led to the defeat of resolutions that would
have implemented that platform. The AMA instead adopted
the policy of boycotting the homeopathists and other sectarians on "ethical," not scientific or educational, grounds. The
idea was to declare all "exclusive dogmas" by definition
unscientific and therefore unethical; conversely, all ethical
practitioners were by implication scientific. The technical
competence of regular and irregular practitioner alike was
to go unexamined.

The failure of the New York State Society and its support-
ers, such as the medical societies in South Carolina and Ohio,
to dominate the AMA in part explains its opposition.[69] In
this regard, ethics came under attack, but not because the
members of the New York Society wanted to associate with
homeopathists. Nor did the New York Society actually
oppose restrictionism, the beginning core for any trade union,
for it was actively working for state licensing to eliminate
incompetents. At issue was the basis on which restriction
would occur and by which institutional means. The New
York Society preferred technical competence determined by
written examination over allegiance to "regular" medical
societies as the basis for restriction, and preferred state
licensure over medical-society ethics as the institutional
means of exclusion.

Ethics could eliminate competitors only if the public
accepted the reputability of the ethical declarations of the
AMA and regular medical societies. Ethics, however, could
not overcome public preference for homeopathist or other
nonorthodox practitioners. The solution was to circumvent
hostile public opinion by creating European-style medical
schools, state licensure, and state boards to administer exam-
that would be controlled by the local regular medical societies. The factions within the regular medical societies that
opposed this solution were those members of poor scientific
merit who relied on their ethical standing for professional

[69] *Ibid.*, p. 176.

status, those who feared the introduction of homeopathist or other well-educated sectarians who could pass state examinations that would be controlled by the local regular medical societies. The factions within the regular medical societies that opposed this solution were those members of poor scientific merit who relied on their ethical standing for professional status, those who feared the introduction of homeopathist or other well-educated sectarians who could pass state examinations, and of course the low-quality, often rural, medical schools. Yet even a well-educated committee from Harvard Medical School headed by Oliver Wendell Holmes opposed the solution, because it believed the emphasis on more education by lecturing a misguided attempt to replace the apprenticeship system.[70] Within two decades, state by state, the position of the New York State Society came to prevail over these objections, and licensure became the principal means for eliminating external competitors in, the United States.

In retrospect, the would-be monopolists on both sides in this dispute appear to have been mistaken. The New York group was surely correct when it held licensing superior to ethics for dealing with irregular practitioners, for licensing is a surer device for suppressing external competitors who might otherwise win public sympathy. But it was mistaken when it tried to eliminate ethical controls over the profession, for it ignored the multiple monopolistic uses of medical ethics: ordering physician conduct and legitimizing the profession's privileges. Both ethical controls and licensure seem to be more effective tools for monopolization in combination than alone. The contemporary persistence of both ethics and licensure bears out the complementary roles which they have played.

Recapitulation

What have I done? I have *not* tried to argue that medical ethics have not helped protect or further the medical interests of patients; clearly, in some respects they probably have

[70] *Ibid.*, pp. 172-173, 176.

helped, yet one would not be very surprised to find ways in which they have hurt patient's interests. But such questions have not been the object of this chapter. I *have* asked how medical ethics have related to the interests of physicians. I have *not* tried to infer the intent of the creators of medical ethics, and I have *not* taken manifest explanations for ethics at face value; I *have* assumed that the creators of medical ethics were aware of the possibility of monopolization when they wrote monopolistic ethics. Having made this assumption, I examined Percival's medical ethics and found that most were latently monopolistic, and then found that their mode of action was to subordinate personal interests of practitioners to the collective interests of the profession and to build collective solidarity. They were able to do so as status conventions, which compensated immediate economic losses with honorific rewards.

I then studied pre-Percivalean ethics and found that documents bearing the name medical ethics had served a variety of organizational ends and that Percival's ethics were comparatively more monopolistic than most. I also found a close similarity between Percival's ethics and the ethics of the Royal College of Physicians of London, and proposed that Percivalean ethics were probably most important for extending the monopolistic strategy of the Royal College of Physicians to other types of privileged practitioners as well.

Having established that monopolization has been only one type of organizational end for medical ethics, I examined in detail the ethics of the American Medical Association and found that medical ethics can serve monopolistic ends in a variety of ways. I found, however, that considerations of public receptivity to the profession's monopolization probably have increasingly influenced medical ethics in recent years, and realized that these pressures have created strain on the system of ethics. Ethics have been used to help order the conduct of physicians in a monopolistic direction, but they have also been used to help make the profession appear less monopolistic for a variety of political reasons. The adoption of dual sets of medical ethics in recent years may help relieve the tension created by this contradiction.

I also found that medical ethics have only limited value as a tool for monopolization. While they are appropriate for ordering the conduct of physicians, redefining the organization of the profession as nonmonopolistic, and legitimizing licensing privileges, they are not appropriate for eliminating external competition.

The following two chapters will examine licensure in England and the United States in historical perspective. The English case is important because the medical profession gained early legal privileges of monopolization and then lost some of these privileges over the centuries. The American case is the opposite: the medical profession gained legal privileges of monopolization late, even though there had been a transient period of early privileges that were weakly monopolistic. While licensure in each case was relatively effective in eliminating external competition, I shall show that licensure, and the struggles over it, played multiple monopolistic roles, much as medical ethics had. It shall also be seen that the study of licensure takes one further into the interest constellations of the medical profession in society, which this study of medical ethics has begun.

CHAPTER FOUR

English Licensure and Monopolization

The preceding study of medical ethics began with the concept of interest-group monopolization from the vantage point of the interest group. Medical ethics can be an organizational tool for organizing physicians for monopolization; nevertheless, this concept alone is inadequate, for successful monopolization requires more than organizing for monopolization. The purpose of this chapter is to investigate the reciprocal side of a monopolization strategy: the political context in which monopolization occurs. The study has suggested already that antimonopolistic legislation is an important political constraint, and this theme and the more general theme of antimonopolistic ideologies will be addressed repeatedly in this chapter and the chapter on American licensure. My task is to find out more about society's receptivity to monopolization efforts, and licensure will serve as an investigative tool. My main concern, therefore, is not actually with licensure per se but with the complex of interests and beliefs with which a monopolizing interest group must deal. Since this confrontation between society and profession is an interaction, I will also inquire into how the medical profession has altered its monopolization strategy in the face of social constraints.

Licensing and the legally privileged group

Licensure is a legal device for classifying members of society into categories according to qualifications. In the case of the medical profession, it usually distinguishes professionals from nonprofessionals, but in some countries such as England it also distinguishes levels of professionals within the medical profession Associated with licensing are specific requirements, privileges and rights reserved for licensees, and penalties for those who infringe upon or illegally assume professional status. Licensing is the legal expression of the principle that renderers of social services should receive special privileges and exemption from normal social regulations. The rise of professions in modern society, particularly over the past two centuries, has based its ascent on social acceptance of this belief. The medical profession's argument has consisted of two parts: licensure is necessary to protect the public from medical practice by unskilled and untrained persons, whether domestics or pretenders, and the performance of medical tasks requires special exemption of the profession from control by many of the legal and moral norms that govern the rest of social life. Such has been the conventional meaning of licensure.

I shall not be concerned with these functional aspects of licensure for the interests of patients. What interests me is that licensing also constitutes the legal basis for the existence of a Weberian "legally privileged group." Legal restriction of activities to only particular persons is by definition monopolistic and helps bring about actual monopolization to the degree that the state enforces the privileges that it guarantees. Therefore, licensing, though conventionally accepted as a means for furthering the public interest, also offers monopolistic benefits for the profession. Indeed, it is not surprising to find in the history of medical licensure that licensing typically has not arisen on the part of nonprofessionals interested in protecting public interests but at the request of professional groups seeking legal privileges. Protection of the public's medical interests has not often been pushed independently by those outside the profession; outsiders have frequently even questioned the public-interest value of medical monopolization on the basis of the profession's eagerness to receive privileges. Hence, the monopolistic aspects of licensure have historically been controversial political issues, which deserve as much theoretical attention as strictly functionalist issues.

I shall address several questions using the concept of the legally privileged group. On what basis did the medical profession acquire legal privileges? How does this basis compare with those of other legally privileged groups contemporaneous with its formation? How did the medical profession try to safeguard its acquired legal privilege and how did it deal with competitors who tried to share in its legal privilege? How did the medical profession come to terms with powerful antimonopolistic political groups, and why did it comply willingly with certain losses of legal privilege? How did these losses affect the monopolization status of the medical profession, and how have they changed the profession's monopolization strategy?

The creation of the Royal College of Physicians

The rise of the Royal College of Physicians of London (RCP) is very important, because of the major role which its struggle for institutionalization and legal privilege has played in the creation of the modern concept of the medical profession. It was primarily a licensing body chartered by King Henry VIII that placed authority for determining who would legally practice medicine into the hands of medical practitioners. As such, it represented a number of historical firsts: the first historical instance of licensing of physicians by a purely professional body—not by church, state, or the universities—and the first institutional example of the medical profession as a distinctively privileged social group and not as an aggregate of prestigious individuals. It also first embodied the modern concept of the medical profession as a body of more-or-less self-regulating medical *practitioners,* who assumed authority on the basis of the claim that practitioners know best how medicine should be practiced and how medical affairs should be conducted.

Professional status has not always been reserved for practitioners. As a means for identifying professional status, licenses had been used in medieval times in such a way as to give "profession" a different meaning. Most European countries during the Middle Ages regarded university degrees as licenses; licensed doctors from the great medical schools of Bologna and Padua, for example, were able to borrow the prestige of the universities situated there. Implicitly, these arrangements implied that licensure certifies acquired education. But, according to this concept, the licensed professional was a seeker of medical truth, not a practitioner. These education licenses often distinguished those with intellectual interests in medicine from those with good intuitive medical skill. This system of licensure predated the modern belief that medical education is necessary for good medical practice, and so whatever prestige the licensed practitioner might have had in the universities and at court was determined by these educational licenses and not by quality of practice. Moreover, licensed doctors did not make their living from practice but from teaching, either through student fees or local-town salaries.[1] The concept of the profession, therefore, was inseparable from the sphere of the universities; the profession was but one type of academic existence and not an independent social group.

The RCP was not merely another guild. To understand the distinction, one should try to place the RCP in comparative context with somewhat dissimilar types of legally privileged social organizations. Weber's description of the general sociological characteristics of the European guilds well suffices for this purpose. The guilds, according to him, were urban combinations of local tradesmen united together for three purposes: mutual help and protection, monopolization of trade rights, and expansion of the economic interests of the guild.[2]

These had by no means been primarily created for the purpose of influencing political conditions. Originally

[1] Vern L. Bullough, *The Development of Medicine as a Profession* (New York: Hafner Publishing Company, 1966), pp. 60-68.

[2] Cf. Max Weber, *Economy and Society: An Outline of Interpretive Sociology*, eds, Guenther Roth and Claus Wittich, 3 vols. (New York: Bedminster Press, 1968), pp. 1252-1253, for a comparison of the guilds with the confraternities of local urban landowners. The landowners' struggles for power differed somewhat from those of the tradesmen, in that the existence of a more or less autonomous city was at stake.

they were substitutes for something their members frequently very much missed in the early medieval city: the backing of a clan, and its protective guarantees. They provided the services otherwise supplied by the clan: help in case of personal injury or threats, aid in economic distress, elimination of feuds between members by means of peaceful conciliation and payment of the wergild liabilities of members (in an English case). The guilds provided for the members' social needs by holding periodic feasts—a practice traceable to pagan ritual meals—and for his funeral with the participation of the breathren; they guaranteed salvation of his soul through good deeds and secured for him from the common treasury indulgences and the benevolence of powerful saints. It goes without saying that such protective associations also represented joint interests, including economic interest.[3]

The English companies resembled the continental urban guilds but not the continental colleges and companies. The members of the English companies "had an exclusive right, conferred by the municipal authorities, of making or selling some particular kind of goods in the civic market and within a specified distance from it."[4] Certain types of medical practitioners also commonly had companies in London from medieval times. Most were separate, such as the companies of the Grocers, the Druggists, the Apothecaries, the Barbers, and the Surgeons. Some formed major multiple-function companies, such as the Barber-Surgeons. A number of practitioners also belonged to more than one company, so that surgeon-apothecaries and other combinations were found.[5] These companies typically had licensing rights, but this similarity should not lead to the false conclusion that the RCP was merely another company or guild.

To better understand the difference, one can use Weber's

[3] *Ibid.*, p. 1256.
[4] Sir George Clark, *A History of the Royal College of Physicians of London,* 2 vols. (Oxford: Clarendon Press for the Royal College of Physicians, 1964, 1966), p. 7.
[5] *Ibid.*, pp. 8-12.

distinction between crafts and craft guilds (*Gilden* and *Zünfte*). These were two types of urban legally privileged groups: the guilds for retail trade and the craft guilds for production (including artisans and others who worked with their hands).[6] The English apothecaries originated in the trade guild of the Company of Grocers, originally dealing in imported spices and exotic materials. By the time they separated from the Company of Grocers in 1620 to form "the Master, Wardens and Society of the Art and Mystery of Apothecaries," the apothecaries had taken on more of the character of a craft guild in that they made and compounded medicines as well as traded in them. The surgeons belonged to craft guilds, since by cutting they employed manual skills. In England and on most of the Continent, surgeons were part of a larger craft guild, the Barber-Surgeons, but occasionally made use of the power of other large craft guilds. In Amsterdam in the sixteenth century the surgeons were in the guild of the makers of wooden shoes. The surgeons frequently tried to improve their own monopolistic position by breaking from the barbers to form their own craft guild, but for various reasons could not do so in England until relatively late.[7]

The English physicians differed from the surgeons and apothecaries in a number of important respects. Despite an abortive attempt in 1423-1424 to form an association of physicians in London, no company (guild or craft guild) of physicians had ever been formed. Physicians neither dealt in trade nor employed manual skills as did the apothecaries and surgeons. Nor did they provide apprenticeships as did guild masters. They were considered educated, not skilled, men. But even though educated in universities, with few exceptions, physicians were usually not members of the faculties of universities.[8] Prior to 1511, they possessed no monopolistic rights; apothecaries and surgeons dispensed advice as well as goods and services, since they did not infringe on any group's guild right by giving advice. The

[6] Weber, *op. cit.*, pp. 1257, 1282.
[7] Clark, *op. cit.*, pp. 6, 9, 12-13, 224.
[8] *Ibid.*, p. 16.

monopolization strategy of the English physicians was to secure monopolistic privileges, the legitimate claim of anyone engaged in gainful activities during medieval times, without sacrificing the traditional prestige of educated status by forming guilds or craft guilds, marked by the inferior prestige of the commercial trades and manual arts. Their solution was to form a unique prestigious corporate body to lay monopolistic claim on the provision of medical advice. They had already gained authority to supervise apothecaries to the King by the time of Edward IV and by 1497 had succeeded in issuing licenses to at least one surgeon on the basis of examination by physicians.[9]

In 1511, Parliament issued an Act restricting the practice of "physick" to those who had been examined by ecclesiastical authorities. It specifically called upon the Bishop of London or the Dean of St. Paul's with the aid of four physicians to examine candidates for a license to practice within the City of London and a seven-mile radius; in the provinces the examination could be performed within a diocese without the presence of physicians.[10] No administrative apparatus was set up to implement this act, however, until 1518 when Thomas Linacre, personal physician to Cardinal Wolsey, and six others petitioned Henry VIII for the creation of a Royal College of Physicians. Ostensibly, the status of the charter was royal and not urban because of the imminent threat to the King of plague, which was epidemic.[11] Evidently, the King's fear of illness had created a favorable political constellation for the creation of the Royal College of Physicians. In any event, the petition was granted, creating a new type of administrative body.

The discontinuity of the Royal College of Physicians with the guild system is also consistent with the use of the term "college" rather than "company" or "mistery." In England, "college" ordinarily meant no more than an "assemblage" of persons, and its administrative use had been restricted to the residential colleges of Oxford and Cambridge and of

9 Ibid., p. 18.
10 Ibid., pp. 54-56.
11 Ibid., p. 58.

the "canons attached to some of the cathedrals and other churches."[12] While this combination of ecclesiastic and academic allusions may have been seized upon as a means for maintaining the distinctive status superiority of physicians in the formation of their mutual association society, there were foreign allusions as well in the word "college." In Florence and Siena, for instance, *collegio* referred to the physician's guild. The French *collèges* were administrative bodies for reviewing licenses in towns without universities; they did not issue licenses but restricted practice only to those with licenses from specific universities.[13] In Flanders, Brabant, and the Low Countries, the administrative representatives of the burgher strata were organized into separate "colleges" to confront appointed counts with local claims.[14]

Since the Royal charter of 1518 refers to the superior management of medical matters abroad,[15] this choice of terms may have been an attempt to appear contemporaneous with foreign developments. Whatever its origin, the word "college" signified in several respects an administrative break from the tradition of the regulative bodies of the European urban guilds and craft guilds. First, the College was an instrument of the interests of the Crown, not of the urban strata. Second, unlike in France where the influence of the University of Paris followed royal consolidation of the provinces,[16] the authority of the RCP was independent of the universities. Third, unlike even the French *collèges*, the Royal College issued its own licenses; it was not a body for checking on the possession of university licenses. Fourth, the Royal College of Physicians claimed the right to imprison as well as prosecute violators of its privileges. This claim was upheld as late as 1602 but rejected with increasing frequency by the courts in later decisions.[17] Fifth, unlike guild members, licentiates of the RCP did not enjoy strictly monopolistic privileges, since other bodies were permitted to issue licenses

[12] *Ibid.*, p. 27.
[13] *Ibid.*, pp. 64, 66.
[14] Weber, *op. cit.* (n. 2, above), p. 1255.
[15] Clark, *op. cit.* (n. 4, above), p. 59.
[16] Bullough, *op. cit.* (n. 1, above), p. 69.
[17] Clark, *op. cit.* (n. 4, above), p. 156.

to practice. The episcopal licensing system persisted into the eighteenth century, despite attempts by the RCP to restrain and eventually eliminate it by law. Also, some university degrees were deemed licenses: graduates of Oxford or Cambridge could practice medicine as physicians anywhere outside the seven-mile radius around London and, later, Westminster. Few, however, did so.[18] Sixth, the Royal College was created as a liturgical arm of the Crown. Its resemblance to a guild, due to their common internal structure of self-government, should not obscure the general difference between their political relationships to outside authorities. A guild used the collective power generated by mutual association and protection as a means of bargaining concessions from urban and sometimes royal authorities.[19]

The Royal College was something new: self-government at the King's command. The monarch's obligation to fulfill certain regulative functions was placed in the hands of a mutual association group, not in ministerial hands. This liturgical relationship to the King gave the Royal College the right to request directly to the Crown for whatever powers it deemed necessary to meet its duty. Petitioning,

---

[18] *Ibid.*, pp. 76, 305.

[19] Weber, *op. cit.* (n. 2, above), p. 1258. With respect to the political role of the urban guilds, Weber writes: "The effect of all these associations was essentially indirect. They facilitated the city union by habituating the burghers to the formation of coalitions in the pursuit of common interests, and of providing models for the cumulation of leadership positions in the hands of persons who had gained experience and social influence in the direction of such association."

Even more to the point, the guilds represented the interests of the burghers against the monarch and the honoratiores. "The patrician families monopolizing the council seats could everywhere maintain this closure easily only as long as no strong contrast of interests arose between them and the excluded part of the citizenry. But once such conflicts emerged, or once the self-esteem of the outs, based on growing wealth and education, and their economic dispensability for administrative work had risen to the point where they could no longer tolerate the idea of being excluded from power, the makings of new revolutions were at hand. Their agents were once again sworn burgher unions, but behind these new unions stood—at times directly identical with them—the craft guilds (*Zünfte*).

"The variable success of the 'craft' revolutions could in extreme cases lead, as we shall see, to a composition of the council exclusively of representatives of the craft guilds and to the typing of full citizenship to membership in one of the 'crafts'. Only this rise of the 'crafts' signified the real seizure of power, or at least general participation in the rule, of the 'bourgeois' classes in the economic sense of the term. Wherever 'craft'-rule (*Zunftherrschaft*) was installed at all effectively, this coincided with the peak of the city's internal power and its greatest internal political independence." Weber, *op. cit.* (n. 2, above), pp. 1281-1282.

not guild bargaining, was established as the RCP's legitimate means for securing group benefits.

So, in a variety of ways, the RCP bore little resemblance to the guilds other than tending toward self-regulation and being a legally privileged group. These differences might be explained by examining how the RCP as a legally privileged group served the interests of physicians. The RCP as a professional group claimed higher prestige than the guild, partly because of the higher prestige of the training of its members in universities but also because of its close and favored position with respect to the Crown. Hence, the Royal College won mostly prestige gains for the physicians. It did not attempt to regulate the behavior of large numbers of physicians: its initial membership was six, increased to twelve by 1522, and to eighteen by 1538.[20] The size of the College did not change until much later, and even then remained a very small body compared to the number of practitioners at large; the use of oral and later written examinations did not mean that the College admitted everyone who passed the examinations. In 1555, the size of the College was set up by statute at twenty, and raised to thirty-four in 1618.[21]

The early members of the Royal College were probably wealthy men, and in any event would have probably better profited economically by spending their time building larger personal practices.[22] Significantly, the College did not publicize its rights or existence but paradoxically regarded as paramount the elimination of "quacks," a task at which it was ineffectual because of its small size, the large number of quacks, and the resistance of the courts.[23] Apparently, and here I speculate, the Royal College had been conferred the prestige of monopolistic access to the royal family and other important people who would have been familiar with laws or had contact with legal advisors. By demanding both a virtual legal monopoly and a small membership, the College showed little concern that its legal privileges forced the

[20] Clark, *op. cit*, (n. 4, above), pp. 70-71.
[21] *Ibid.*, pp. 132, 188, 517.
[22] *Ibid.*, p. 64.
[23] *Ibid.*, p. 148.

masses to seek illegal medical advice. In general, it cared very little for the state of the profession in the provinces outside London. Though it insisted that all licensed physicians travel to London for examination as "extra-licentiates," it admitted only about eighty provincial practitioners between 1691 and 1750, and did not prosecute any provincial violators, though still retaining the right to do so.[24] Thus, the professional body was likely using licensure as a means for maintaining its collective presence at court.

Yet it also attempted to prosecute violators from time to time who had not had anything to do with the royal court. In light of the frank inability of the College to discipline and police these violators, it would appear that the claim to the right to discipline was more important for the justification of the privileges of the College than for the fulfillment of functional purposes for society.

Safeguarding monopolistic privilege

So far I have examined the creation of the modern concept of the profession, following how the rise of monarchical power in England made possible a break from medieval guild traditions. With a royal charter for a new type of privileged group, the Royal College of Physicians brought into being a new concept of the profession: practitioners instead of academics. This group was not yet privileged by statutory law, for it had only a royal charter, that is, it existed only at the King's command. While licensure for physicians was already statutory law, the corporate existence of the RCP was not. The institutional problem which the early RCP thus faced was that the Crown might remove its charter if its members fell into royal disfavor. The strategy which the RCP followed was to dissociate its institutional fate as much as possible from royal arbitrariness. This strategy was two-fold: transformation from a patrimonially to a legislatively privileged group through typification, and redefinition of professional service in an autonomous direction.

Weber uses the term "typification" for the conversion of

---

[24] *Ibid.*, pp. 77, 140, 519-520, 537-538.

monarchical benefices and other privileged offerings into righful legal possessions by the beneficiaries.[25] The Royal College typified its gains when the members of the new profession turned to Parliament in 1523 for an act to secure its royal charter under statutory law.[26] Yet, in trying to typify its gains, it brought into question the status of its liturgical relationship to the King. If the Royal College were no longer to serve the purposes of the Crown, how could it legitimize its continued existence, in possible opposition to the King's will, no less? Because physicians provided care for many important political figures, they had little practical difficult in obtaining Parliamentary support. The hard problem was to justify legislative legalization of the RCP's privileged position. Such legalization was finally legitimized by redefining service in a politically favorable way.

The RCP's solution was to associate itself with the idea of national service, a concept emerging with the strengthening of Parliament, itself a typified institution. Along these lines, the 1523 Act included new provisions to reflect this new basis for legitimation. It required for the first time that no one should practice as a physician anywhere *in England* without examination in London by the President of the College and three "elects."[27] Only graduates of Cambridge or Oxford were entitled to become provincial physicians without examination before the College. Such examination of provincial physicians had not been provided for in the Act of 1511. Yet the distinction between licentiates, who had to be examined before the College to practice in the London area, and the extra-licentiates, who could be excused from examination by holding an "Oxbridge" degree, was founded on the separation of the jurisdiction of London from that of the provinces. In this sense, the College did not claim to provide uniform service to the nation; but its claim of the right to license nation-wide, except in special cases, represented a change in the profession's ideology. Typification by Parliament had freed the College from its liturgical

[25] Weber, *op. cit.* (n. 2, above), p. 1012.
[26] Clark, *op. cit.* (n. 4, above), pp. 75-76.
[27] *Ibid.*, p. 77.

status vis-à-vis the King by substituting a more abstract, impersonal duty to "England." The void of this undefined duty was filled by the Royal College with the creation of the concept of professional authority. It was henceforth the duty of the profession to use its education in an unspecified manner to determine medical problems, find solutions, and implement them. The Royal College succeeded in this way in monopolizing the right to define its own national duty. If necessary, it would reject the King's bidding in favor of what it believed best on the basis of its expertise. This authority did not extend in guild fashion only to a town but was coextant with the kingdom, i.e., the sphere of monarchical domination.

In the long run, this ideological change in behalf of typification has been more important than the legal privileges themselves for the shaping of the modern concept of the profession. The self-regulatory right to license group members continues into the present for the English profession but exists in no other nation. Nonetheless, even in those nations where the profession has never gained this right, or even in the United States, where it lost the sporadically-held right, the profession still uses some variation of the professional ideologies which the Royal College created to redefine its relationship to ruling administrative powers. Hence, the idea that national medical service and the right to define it are realms of the profession and of no other authority—a distinctively English idea—has spread to medical professions in other nations even when the English system of licensure has not been adopted.

The RCP, safeguarding its newly won monopolistic privileges, had turned to Parliament for legislative guarantees. In the process, it repudiated certain claims of patrimonial domination and elaborated the ideology that the purposes of the medical profession should be determined only by physicians. The 1523 Act deleted the earlier requirements for ecclesiastical participation in medical licensing and so gave the profession a secular character by removing religious authorities from medical policy making. It also freed the profession from its liturgical relationship to the King. So, even while the name Royal College of Physicians indicated the patrimonial nature of the profession's origins, the group's power struggles with the Church and the Crown changed the political basis of the profession's monopolistic privileges and of the ideologies which legitimized its privileges.

Dealing with external competitors

The 1523 Act greatly furthered the removal of ecclesiastics from medical affairs by placing responsibility for licensing in secular practitioners' hands and not, as *per traditionem,* in religious hands. Yet the Church retained its right to have medical practitioners, so the RCP's legal privileges were monopolistic except for canon law. As secular law gradually triumphed over canon law in everyday life, the RCP's legal privileges became increasingly monopolistic in value. In any event, the most important competitors of the RCP were not clerical. Other practitioners who engaged in activities similar to those of the physicians were also at times interested in acquiring professional rather than guild status. One problem which the RCP faced was the maintenance of superior prestige without bringing into question its own legitimizing ideologies. Another problem was the enforcement of the RCP's legal privileges at a time when the state was both relatively weak and indifferent.

The Royal College had attained higher prestige than the companies of the surgeons and apothecaries by developing a theory of its special qualities and duties and by creating an institutional basis different than the companies. To justify its special privileges, the Royal College claimed that a profession was different from a trade or craft, a belief that still is heard today in England. The Royal College even claimed the right to supervise the quality of the preparations of the apothecaries; no guild had ever had the right to interfere with the regulation of the activities of another guild or to subordinate another. The medieval theory of the legitimate monopolization of trades and crafts by guilds resulted in extensive horizontal differentiation. The Royal College's theory of professional authority provided for both horizontal differentiation in the form of monopolization and vertical differentiation in the form of regulation of the medical guilds, which were deemed inferior to the profession. Not surprisingly, the surgeon and apothecary companies resented and resisted the superior position and domination of the physicians.

One way in which the RCP tried to eliminate its competitors is illustrated by its early treatment of the apothecaries. The apothecaries commonly provided advice, along with the drugs which they prepared and sold, and so intruded on the physicians' legal monopolization on advice. The RCP met this problem by helping the apothecaries create their own guild in 1614, using their influence to help the weak faction of apothecaries break from the Grocer's company. This action was in the interests of the Royal College, or so it appeared at the time. One of the Elects of the College reported that the terms of the agreement between the apothecaries, the grocers, and the physicians included that the apothecaries "be bound by their freeman's oath not to give advice to patients or to offer them service except in emergencies and not to make up prescriptions other than those of physicians recognized by the College."[28] By 1617, the apothecaries were incorporated as a company and royally proclaimed in 1620. After 1684, it went by the name of the Society of Apothecaries.[29] Evidently, the RCP hoped to control competition with the apothecaries by relying on traditional guild regulation to compensate for lack of state enforcement of the group's legal privileges. In exchange for guild status, the apothecaries were expected to honor the RCP's monopolization of advice and not fill competitors' prescriptions, all of which amounted to transforming the apothecaries into servants of the interests of physicians.

This strategy of reducing competition by dominating competitors through guild controls did not work out very well for the physicians. For one thing, the RCP did not work to eliminate illegal practitioners, so the apothecaries felt that the RCP did not support their monopolization claims under the guild system. Moreover, many apothecaries with illegal

[28] *Ibid.*, p. 222.
[29] *Ibid.*, p. 224.

yet technically adequate medical practices regarded the privileges of the physicians as unjustified. This company and the company of surgeons, as well, resented the physicians' superior status claims, particularly since the physicians viewed even surgeons with similar educations at Oxford and Cambridge as inferior. The prestige component was very important, for in time both surgeons and apothecaries found it in their interest to attempt to share in the physicians' prestige by identifying with the concept of the profession that the College had fostered. These groups developed the idea that, since most medical practitioners in England were not physicians, equal licensing privileges should be extended. So the strategy of guild controls resulted in the competition's becoming interested in acquiring legal privileges for itself equal to those of the physicians, instead of continuing with illegal competition. The use of guild controls was probably unrealistic in any event, due to the very large market for medical care and the very small number of physicians; economic opportunities were too great and the regulatory power of the guilds too weak.

The next strategy of the RCP was to accept the movement for licensing privileges for the surgeons and apothecaries but to reject equal privileges. By the end of the eighteenth century, the RCP had become receptive to admitting both surgeons and apothecaries to the medical profession on the condition that the distinctive position of the physicians be maintained.[30] The distinction was maintained in two ways. In 1797 the surgeons, who had succeeded in breaking from the Barber's Company in 1754 by Act of Parliament,[31] received a royal charter for a Royal College of Surgeons at the suggestion of the Royal College of Physicians. Unlike the RCP, this body had no coercive powers but only conducted examinations and issued licenses. The examining committee was formed of fulltime surgeons, who were bound to accept all who passed their examinations.[32] The RCS, then, furthered the RCP's monopolization by providing an equally prestigious license for practitioners of surgery, who would

[30] Ibid., p. 622.
[31] Ibid., p. 596.
[32] Ibid., p. 624.

hopefully not practice in RCP domain. By this means, the RCP hoped to further horizontal differentiation by providing equal status awards for surgeons.

Along a different line, the RCP also supported the conversion of the Society of Apothecaries into an examining body later in 1815. More than the surgeons, the apothecaries had infringed on the RCP's monopolization of advice, but the RCP supported licensing because the apothecaries set lower standards for their license and so preserved the physicians' higher prestige. The RCP made certain that the invidious status of the apothecaries would persist. The apothecaries at the insistence of the Royal College provided for apprenticeship so that the apothecaries' guild origins would not be forgotten. Similarly, the apothecaries were forbidden from charging for advice and had to be satisfied with guildlike income from medications. They accepted these invidious conditions for a variety of reasons. As has been mentioned, they had long been dissatisfied with unlicensed status as medical practitioners, especially since they performed most of the nation's medical practice. More immediately, however, the druggists and chemists had stepped up their competition with the apothecaries, and so the apothecaries safeguarded their interests by submitting to licensure, even if not on equal terms with the physicians.

Not all invidious conditions remained. The apprenticeship requirement was later woven into the curriculum of medical education and so superseded. A court decision of 1811 had permitted fees for advice from apothecaries, and so court decisions subsequent to the Act of 1815 likewise did not uphold the provisions for charges.[33] In this manner, certain status aspirations of the practicing apothecaries and surgeon-apothecaries were satisfied without destroying the higher prestige of the elite of physicians or of the newly created Royal College of Surgeons. So, in effect, licensing the apothecaries under these terms supported the RCP's monopolization by ensuring its status superiority even though strict horizontal differentiation had not been maintained.

[33] *Ibid.*, p. 649.

Clearly, the monopolization strategy of the RCP had changed. No longer did it claim sole legal privilege to medical practice or deny others professional status. Henceforth it claimed elite status within an extended medical profession. In part, this change was on account of the famous Rose decision by the House of Lords in 1703, in which the monopolistic claims of the RCP were rejected, much to the College's surprise. As time passed, the RCP found convictions harder to win from the courts and encountered judicial reluctance to uphold the College's coercive powers. A legal authority in 1834 wrote that the Rose decision appeared "rather to have been produced by feeling than by a strict adherence to the existing law."[34] As far as the courts were concerned, the College could not successfully lay claim to representing the medical profession. If it could not pursue this line of monopolization, it could only hope to establish superiority within the profession. To some degree it successfully established the idea of a vertically structured, conglomerate profession; but in the process it also brought together the support of the surgeons and the apothecaries to bear on another political problem: the developing fight to preserve the principle of licensed professionalism. Ultimately the RCP fought two battles: one for supremacy within the medical profession and another for survival of monopolistic professionalization as an institutional principle. The profession had risen on the shoulders of the medieval principle of monopolistic urban guilds, but when monopolies came under attack by classical liberal philosophers and politicians, the profession had to find new justification for its monopolization. Its earlier battle had been to justify its uniqueness in a social world of legitimate guild monopolies as a monopoly which regulated neither trade nor craft; now it had to establish itself in a more democratic world.

Professional monopolization and the rise of English liberalism

So far I have discussed the creation and rise of an interest group, its attainment of royal and then legislated privileges,

[34] *Ibid.*, p. 479.

and its struggles with competing interest groups. The problem of competition with other medical practitioners was more or less resolved by propagating the concept of the modern profession beyond the boundaries of the RCP. In exchange for professional status, practitioners outside the RCP recognized its relative superiority, but such status differences did not prevent the three professional groups—the physicians, surgeons, and apothecaries—from henceforth presenting a united front to the rest of society. By the beginning of the nineteenth century, a united front was apparently necessary for all three groups because antimonopolistic beliefs became politically salient. My study will now turn to this problem of how the organized medical profession during the nineteenth century—this conglomerate of three semicompetitive interest groups—dealt with the challenge of antimonopolism. The RCP remains important, however, because of its continuing role as an ideological center for the extended medical profession.

One is thus led to inquire into how antimonopolistic beliefs became politically important, how these beliefs threatened the position and institutional stability of the organized medical profession, how the profession modified ideologies to answer the objections of opponents, and finally how it came to terms with these opponents.

Since its inception, the RCP had attempted to establish a place among the English aristocracy on the basis of education. Like aristocrats, physicians possessed a title, even if nonhereditary. They also belonged to a royally and legislatively recognized social group, the College, even though they had passed an examination to enter it. Moreover, like the aristocracy, the medical profession pushed the idea of service to the nation by the higher classes. The medical profession had ideologically and ritualistically emulated the English aristocracy but never shared the same basis of legitimacy for aristocratic status or claimed full entry into the aristocracy. Imitation may have been the sincerest form of flattery in the profession's case, especially since it did not threaten the aristocratic order; but as the middle classes rose to power at the end of the eighteenth century, the profession was pressed to answer critics among the bourgeoisie. Unlike the professions the contemporary entrepreneurial class was attempting to bring about a class revolution in England, which entailed new ideologies to justify subordination and treatment of workers.[35] In the course of power struggles with the aristocracy, the ascendent middle class elaborated principles of moral conduct with which the medical profession had to come to terms. The profession had three choices: identify with the aristocracy, identify with the rising entrepreneurial class, or create a unique identity for the profession in modern society. By extricating itself from the struggle between entrepreneurs and aristocrats, the profession could hope to retain privileges regardless of the outcome.

The entrepreneurial-class philosophers generated three major ideologies which threatened the professional orders: liberalism, libertarianism, and laissez faire. Though all three ideologies might be subsumed under the thought of certain liberal thinkers as "liberalism," for the purposes of this study liberalism will refer to the belief in the social desirability of maximizing economic competition in the marketplace, libertarianism to the belief in the moral desirability of maximizing the freedom of individuals to do as they please, and laissez faire to the belief in the desirability of state nonintervention in economic affairs. Together they present a world image of free-willed, legally unhindered, competing individuals releasing their energy in behalf of unplanned social progress. I shall overlook for most of the rest of this study that these beliefs together contained several contradictions, for the important point is that they were strongly believed in in strategic quarters and that they implied certain consequences for the medical profession as an institution. Yet a brief mention of these contradictions is in order.

To the extent that competition leads to differential success and the concentration of wealth and power into fewer hands, competition undermines the conditions for its own existence. This is because the monopolization process described by Weber is fundamentally a form of competition, only by

[35] Reinhard Bendix, *Work and Authority in Industry* (New York and Evanston: Harper & Row, 1956), pp. 15-17, 101, 115, 441.

organized men. In this sense the logical, even if not empirical, outcome of competition is monopolization of market supply. To prevent organized competition, i.e. monopolization, individuals cannot be permitted to organize for advantage; but prevention compromises economic libertarian rights to do as one pleases and, insofar as a powerful party is necessary for restraint, compromises laissez faire beliefs. Therefore in these senses, liberalism bears a negative relationship to libertarianism and laissez faire. Put more simply, an ongoing competitive market requires some measure of intervention to maintain competitive conditions.

Libertarianism and laissez faire are incompatible in the sense that men free to do as they please may alone or in combination deny each other freedom. Without state or equivalent intervention, libertarianism also logically undermines its own existence by creating the conditions for unfreedom and oppression. Therefore, libertarianism and laissez faire are incompatible in an analogous sense to the incompatibility of liberalism with libertarianism and laissez faire. Yet one may overlook these logical incompatibilities to see the common political purposes to which these beliefs were put in behalf of class interests.

The entrepreneurial class could attack the medical profession on a number of counts. In a letter to a member of the RCP, the political economist Adam Smith found the profession's corporate monopolism unjustifiable.[36] He argued that anyone should be free to practice medicine and that good physicians should be chosen on the basis of the quality of performance ("merit") and not education. His simple argument implies all three anticorporation beliefs. He is a libertarian when he recognizes that any type of licensing constitutes a hindrance to free trade both in terms of supplier freedom and consumer sovereignty. He is a liberal when he implies that physicians should compete for patients on the basis of their reputations of merit. And he is a noninterventionist when he opposes the role of the corporations in licensing physicians and the legally privileged position of

---

[36] Clark, *op. cit.* (n. 4, above), p. 569. Also cf. John Rae, *Life of Adam Smith* (New York: Augustus M. Kelley, 1965 [1895]), pp. 273-280.

licensed physicians. Smith's comments threatened the existing medical profession, then, since he essentially called for an end to licensing and to the profession as a legally privileged group.

The profession's initial strategy was to revive traditional professional ideologies to assert the inapplicability of liberal principles for the medical profession. The only hope for the medical profession was to continue denying that it was a trade. Since libertarian arguments centered on the importance of free trade, they could be circumvented by claiming that the profession did not engage in trade at all. It could also help the interests of the profession to claim that fulfillment of its activities required the corporate privileges under attack. The concepts of service and professional authority therefore again came to the fore. The RCP had distinguished itself from the guilds and craft guilds by declaring itself a profession. It did not produce or trade goods; it issued advice. Since advice was not a trade item or possession, professional services ought not to be regarded as subject to free-trade considerations. The apothecaries and surgeons, from whom the RCP had earlier distinguished itself, were identified with the medical profession by relegating manual skills and, in the case of the apothecaries, trade in drugs to the position of instruments for professional service.

This theme continues today. Carr-Saunder's classic 1933 work on the professions stresses the idea of the professions as different from trades:[37]

Many of the professions, as we have seen, were evolved, directly or indirectly, out of the Church, and they inherited from the Church the ideal of devotion to a calling. These professions reached their full stature and others began to make their appearance at a period when the conception of the "gentleman" was supreme, and from the "gentleman" with whom their members associated they derived other ideals which are no less a part of the professional code. Thus a "gentleman" might be

[37] A. M. Carr-Saunders, and P. A. Wilson, *The Professions* (Oxford: The Clarendon Press, 1933), pp. 420-441.

rich and might even seek riches. But certain roads to
the acquisition of riches were closed to him; in particular
he must not seek riches through the avenue of "trade."[38]

During the negotiations for the creation of the National
Health Service in 1945-47, the British Medical Association
and other health professional associations were "proud of
the fact that they are not trade unions, and that many of
their members would be horrified at being called trade
unionists." In 1871, in an ironic twist of history, trade unions
had been debarred from registration as companies, yet professional associations were so registered.[39] Both ideologically
and institutionally the medical profession succeeded in acquiring recognition as a special case in England. Even the
language of professional business maintained the distinction.
Physicians do not place prices on their services but charge
fees. They have no customers but clients. They do not
advertise or solicit clients. It is not just that the profession
is "above that sort of thing;" they are engaged in service,
not trade.

The antilibertarian service ideologies of the medical profession also implied that the state should intervene through
the medical corporations. If medical services were to be
performed, it was argued, the profit motive had to be tran-
scended, since services were supposedly not motivated by
the desire for profit and so did not come under the umbrella
of the theory of the "invisible hand": the idea that the pursuit
of personal interests redounds to the good of society. The
RCP tried to legitimize its existence by arguing that its main
function was the elimination of quacks to protect the public.[40]
That it had been ineffective at the task did not deter it from
stating that this was its purpose. The RCP did not follow
the argument to the logical conclusion that state intervention beyond the medical corporations would be necessary,
for at least initially in this debate the RCP did not wish
to concede its traditional functions. In this respect, the

[38] *Ibid.*, pp. 420-421.
[39] H. A. Clegg, and T. E. Chester, *Wage Policy and the Health Service* (Oxford:
Basil Blackwell, 1957), p. 11.
[40] Clark, *op. cit.* (n. 4, above), p. 677.

medical profession shared in some of the laissez faire attitudes of the liberal philosophers: it opposed intervention
whenever its own interests were threatened.

Later liberal ideologies developed versions of the idea that
the masses should be self-dependent. The most familiar
version is the idea of *caveat emptor* in the marketplace. No
one and no institution were to be held responsible for the
fate and condition of the unfortunate, for everyone's place
in society was the result of his own conduct.[41] The state
was not to interfere in social matters; to do so would violate
the doctrine of self-help as well as restrict free trade. The
doctrine of *caveat emptor* threatened the medical profession
by calling into question the raison d'être of the medical corporations: elimination of quacks to protect the public. The
profession responded with the exemption argument again and
asserted that *caveat emptor* was not applicable in health
matters. In a letter to Adam Smith, the prominent physician
William Cullen of Edinburgh declared that in medicine "none
of the reasons for unfettered competition are of any force. . . .
The community are scarcely able to judge . . . of the merits
of medical men. . . . The life and health of a great portion
of mankind are in the hands of ignorant people. . . . The
legislatures should take especial care that the necessary art
should, as far as possible, be rendered both safe and useful
to society."[42]

Since the mainstay of Smith's belief that laymen can
rationally obtain medical help through the open market—
reputation—may be based on other attributes than qualified
training, it falls to those with qualified training to identify
those who are qualified, because only they can apply the
critical criteria. Cullen's argument supported the existence
of the medical corporations—and the profession—by legitimizing licensure, the structural feature upon which all the
other legal functions of the corporations have depended.
Within Cullen's ideology, licensing should exist to distinguish
the qualified from the unqualified. Since university degrees

[41] Bendix, *op. cit.*, p. 115.
[42] David L. Cowen, "Liberty, Laissez-Faire and Licensure in Nineteenth Century
Britain," *Bulletin of the History of Medicine* 43 (January-February 1969), p. 31.

were not sufficient evidence of qualification of merit, only
the best men of the profession could decide if a practitioner
were qualified. Essentially, this argument rests on characteristics of dependence imputed to patients; they are depicted
as irrational, ignorant, and incapable of entering the market
as rational individuals. Any alternative to licensing would
permit quacks to exploit the desperation of the sick and
possibly to injure them. Therefore, the doctrine of *caveat
emptor* should not apply to the unusual case of the medical
profession.

The emerging ideology rested increasingly on the construction of a justification of the doctrine of patient dependence. As Bendix has stated, laissez faire doctrines tended
to deny an obligation for the higher classes to care for the
poor. The condition of people was held to be due to their
own efforts and their ability to develop self-dependence. The
original doctrine had referred to the problem of welfare for
the poor, but the profession's traditional commitment to the
Christian principle of gratuitous care for the poor was also
untenable for the liberals. Medical care represented one of
the incentives for hard work; to remove it would weaken
the moral structure of productive society. Yet the term
"self-dependence" could take on an additional meaning. The
emergent professional ideology seized on the idea that the
patient is helpless. The liberals might believe it immoral to
help those who might help themselves, but they would have
a hard time opposing protection of the helpless. If the
self-help doctrine could be suspended for the case of the
medical profession, the profession's activities could be shown
to be nonthreatening to the moral order of the entrepreneurs.

Clearly, the medical profession's political condition did not
correspond well with developing bourgeois ideologies. Licensing and the monopolistic corporations were incompatible
with liberalism, libertarianism, and laissez faire. Smith, for
instance, had argued that patients should be free to select
doctors on the basis of reputation instead of licensing and
that anyone should be free to practice medicine; later laissez
faire theorists argued that the sliding scale removed work
incentives and discouraged the development of consumer

rationality. The medical profession tried to argue that these ideologies did not apply to the special case of the profession. Free trade in medicine is inappropriate, since the profession sells services and not goods. Patients cannot rationally judge reputations because of inadequate knowledge, so they must rely on professional judgments. Moreover, the doctrine of self-help is inappropriate, since the patient is not in a position to increase his rationality. Therefore, the profession argued, monopolistic privileges should be continued.

How adequate were these arguments? On the level of logic, what the organized medical profession had attempted to do was to redefine its activities differently than had the liberals. Its arguments relied on unknowable claims, such as that professionals in fact judge each other more beneficially for the patient than the patient might, and on highly subjective claims, such as that selling services entails motives different from selling goods. Similarly, the low capacity of laymen to acquire adequate rationality in selecting physicians was at best an unverified idea. The profession's claims were thus neither valid nor invalid, and so the liberals were not bound to accept this redefining of the situation. On the level of politics, the organized medical profession did not seem to fare very well with the liberals. By and large, its claims were rejected and its traditional legal privileges revoked. Yet at the same time it acquired new legal privileges which gave the profession a number of potent competitive advantages. Thus, it is not very surprising to find that the medical profession for the most part supported certain institutional changes which stripped it of its old privileges.

Settling with the bourgeoisie: new legal privileges for old

The clash with the liberals was not resolved until the medical profession underwent a number of institutional changes in 1858. The Medical Act of 1858 is interesting theoretically, since it changed medical licensing practices in a way consistent with liberal thought and inconsistent with the profession's traditional monopolization strategy. The Medical Act removed legal restrictions on medical practice, permitting anyone to practice who wished to, but maintained the medical corporations' privilege to issue licenses. Those with legal licenses were listed in an official *Medical Register,* which was regulated along with the licensing corporations through a General Medical Council (GMC) ultimately responsible to the Privy Council. The GMC was empowered to remove licensed practitioners from the *Medical Register* under certain circumstances and to refuse to accept licenses from corporations which did not meet minimal examination standards. Once licensed, however, a practitioner always retained his license unless revoked by the corporation, even if he were stricken from the *Medical Register.* While anyone was free to practice medicine, only those in the *Medical Register* could sue for fees or be employed by the state.

No longer was the medical profession a legally privileged group in the earlier sense. It did not legally restrict practice only to members of the interest group, did not exercise sole control over entry into the group, and did not prosecute competitors. As early as 1840, in fact, the Royal College of Physicians had finally relinquished all matters dealing with prosecution to the "Civil Magistrate."[43] The RCP declined to prosecute for several reasons. For one thing, it could not do so effectively. The medical corporations lacked adequate administrative machinery, and the courts refused to honor prosecutions. For another, the liberals had raised questions about English rights of liberty that the profession had to handle gingerly. In practical terms, libertarian sentiment was older and more universal in England and hence more important than liberalism. Even if the public could not judge physicians adequately to make possible rational competition, there was some question whether the state had the right to prevent free men from engaging in free trade. Yet free trade did not imply state nonintervention. These new laws of 1858 provided for an unprecedented participation of the English government in medical affairs and gave the state a number of functions where the profession had previously been autonomous, such as setting standards for licensing, punishing violators by revoking formal recognition, and officially designating approved practitioners.

[43] Clark, *op. cit.* (n. 4, above), p. 702.

Yet one should not conclude that the organized medical profession was less monopolistic: its monopolization strategy had only changed to accommodate differences with liberal critics. The profession, despite these institutional changes, was still able to push its own interests. These institutional changes apparently redounded to the interests of the profession in four ways. They helped maintain the institutional existence of the medical corporations and licensing, stabilized internal relations among professional bodies, used state recognition in new ways to give licensed practitioners a competitive advantage, and disarmed liberal attacks.

Most important for the medical profession, the continued existence and function of the licensing bodies had been guaranteed. This guarantee was a substantial gain, since liberal ideologies proposed that licensing bodies, as agents of monopoly, ought to be done away with. The creation of the GMC did not really supersede the medical corporations, for the task of the GMC was primarily to register licenses from the corporations. Nor did apparent state intervention greatly compromise the domination of the corporations. Despite formal supervision of the GMC by the Privy Council, the GMC was composed predominantly of professionals. Nine representatives were from the medical corporations, eight from the universities, and six nominated by the Crown.[44] On the basis of expertise, the representatives from the corporations tended to assert authority for policy-making and to make the GMC a legal tool of the interests of the corporations. In this light, the net effect of the 1858 Act was to give the medical corporations a new political tool for pursuing their interests, a far cry from doing away with the corporations althogether.

One remarkable fact about the 1858 Act and the GMC was that they pleased all participants, particularly the medical corporations. One reason for this was that they helped stabilize relationships among the corporations, which had been turbulent because of lingering resentments and jealousies. The Royal Colleges preserved their status privileges by listing the individual qualifications of all registrants in the

[44] W. L. Burn, *The Age of Equipoise* (New York: W. W. Norton & Company, 1964), pp. 202-211.

Medical Register; therefore, the prestige value of a license from the Royal Colleges could be publicized through the official register. The reforms also pleased the apothecaries. The general practitioners, a term for apothecaries practicing both medicine and surgery which arose during the twenty years following the Apothecaries' Act of 1815, had formed a national self-protective association in 1832 (the Provincial Medical and Surgical Association, renamed the British Medical Association in 1856). They had originally set legislative machinery in motion by appealing for medical reform in 1839—reform in this context referring to the extension of privileges to lower classes of practitioners, not to the modern meaning of upgrading quality. The reformers failed to eliminate privileges by abolishing the corporations and instead received equal rights and privileges though perhaps not equal status. They could practice anywhere in Great Britain; the medical profession had abandoned the medieval system of separate territorial jurisdictions for each medical order.

Most important, any registered practitioner, regardless of the type of license he held, could sue for fees and be employed in public service.[45] So even if the general practitioner did not enjoy equal prestige with the physician, he was henceforth permitted to do anything that the physician might and to share in equal rights. These gains for the lower medical order helped at least for a while in easing internal strain and competition within the profession.

The new system of licensing did not entirely cease its competitive value for the medical profession. To be sure, licensing no longer prohibited outsiders from practicing medicine, but it provided competitive value in at least three other ways.

First, licensing gave registered practitioners a psychological advantage over others by providing them with apparent state approval; that is, the prestige of the state was thrown behind members of the organized medical profession. The prospective patient might be more likely to select a state-approved practitioner than one with only a good community or professional reputation for a number of more or less

[45] *Ibid.*

irrational reasons, such as the belief that the state would
not authorize poor physicians or the belief that the state
had independently evaluated practitioners and was not self-
interested like the medical corporations. Also, state approval
simply set off registered practitioners as a group from unregistered practitioners, strongly implying that the most important choice was between these two groups and not among
individual practitioners. Medical licensing examinations
were not like merit examinations of the type arising during
the Victorian period. The Victorian merit examination, when
it appeared a generation later, would fill administrative
positions on the basis of written examinations. Merit would
be redefined as the ranked score of an applicant on a technical
examination, not the possession of formal degrees (though
these might be prerequisites for application), and certainly
not quality performance of practice. These merit examinations, like the liberals, would encourage competition among
individuals in the belief that it would lead to excellence,
but in this instance, through competition for bureaucratic
offices.[46]

The medical examinations served a different goal. Though
the state also seemingly encouraged competition among
medical students for entry into the profession, the examinations were part of the emergent idea of the "safe, general
practitioner," which arose about 1861.[47] The idea corresponded with the structural fact that members of the profession were not ranked along a scale of offices as in bureaucratic
structures but were either in or out of the profession on
an all-or-none basis. Medical examinations, therefore, tended
to pass over the relative quality of applicants in order to
test for applicants not worthy of entrance into the profession.
The profession's traditional emphasis since medieval times
on the difference between the qualified and unqualified
practitioner encouraged this development, even though the
examinations were criticized because of their emphasis on
exclusion. The argument against them claimed that a focus

[46] *Ibid.*, pp. 141-142.
[47] Charles Newman, *The Evolution of Medical Education in the Nineteenth
Century* (London: Oxford University Press, 1957), p. 203.

on exclusion rather than placement of applicants favored the development of mediocre, uniform standards, not qualities of mind that could individuate the best doctors. One observer, Newman, states that the examinations encouraged students to become safe doctors, not good doctors.[48] The point is that medical examinations were used essentially for licensed practitioners to compete with unlicensed practitioners and not for intraprofessional competition.

Second, the state tended to increase what economists would today call the marginal utility of a licensed practitioners' services by legally guaranteeing the quality of licenses. The GMC was empowered to review the standards and questions of the licensing corporations and could refuse to accept an inadequate license, though it never did so. Perhaps licensing standards were always found adequate because of the policing effects of the GMC, but one should also remember that the GMC required medical experts to evaluate the quality of the examinations and gave the task to the elites of the licensing bodies. In this case as in general with the GMC, an institution which appeared to the public to evaluate licenses disinterestedly was controlled in fact by the same group it was supposed to regulate. Yet regardless of who really exercised control, governmental minimal standards for licensing increased the market value of licensed services. Even the liberal philosopher and former physician T.H. Huxley qualified laissez faire beliefs by admiring the benefits of state review of licensing standards:

> It is now, I am sorry to say, something over forty years since I began my medical studies, and, at that time, the state of affairs was extremely singular ... At that time, there were twenty-one licensing bodies—that is to say, bodies whose certificate was received by the State as evidence that the persons who possessed that certificate were medical experts. ... They were partly universities, partly medical guilds and corporations, partly the Archbishop of Canterbury. There was no central authority, there was nothing to prevent any one of these

[48] *Ibid.*, p. 200.

licensing authorities from granting a license to anyone upon any conditions it thought fit. The examination might be a sham, the curriculum might be a sham, the certificate might be bought and sold like anything in a shop; or, on the other hand, the examination might be fairly good and the diploma correspondingly valuable; but there was not the smallest guarantee, except the personal character of the people who composed the administration of each of these licensing bodies, as to what might happen. It was possible for a young man to come to London and to spend two years and six months of the time of his compulsory three years "walking the hospitals" in idleness or worse; he could then by putting himself in the hands of a judicious "grinder" for the remaining six months, pass triumphantly through the ordeal of one hour's *viva voce* examination, which was all that was absolutely necessary, to enable him to be turned loose upon the public, like Death on the pale horse, "conquering and to conquer," with the full sanction of the law, as a "qualified practitioner."[49]

Third, the licensed medical profession was given a new legal privilege: a monopoly on state employment. Partly this right was reserved by the 1858 Medical Act because of the belief that the state could employ only those whom it officially recognized, for constitutionally the state did not share in the liberty rights of Englishmen regarding free trade. While this right did not give the medical profession a competitive advantage in the open market, it monopolized a sector of the market: state services. As will be seen, it also had a potential capacity for helping the profession monopolize the open market, but that potential would not be realized for almost another century.

The new licensing institutions also helped disarm liberal attacks. As has been seen, even the prominent liberal Huxley approved of them. How did they deal with the antagonistic ideologies? Previously, as I have discussed, the organized

---

[49] T. H. Huxley, "The State and the Medical Profession," *Nineteenth Century* 15 (1884), pp. 230-231.

medical profession had tried to exempt itself from the terms of liberal theory by asserting its inapplicability in this special case. While some of the arguments were thought-provoking, they were not conclusive and were not sufficient to break down the relatively closed ideological system of the liberals. The new institutional changes, on the contrary, were interpretable by the profession in terms compatible with liberal theory.

The organized profession had turned the tables on the liberals and used Adam Smith's arguments against them. Since licensing would have ensured the existence of the corporations, the profession suggested a rationale for licensing that would please liberals. According to Adam Smith, the profession should maintain itself on the strength of the merit of its practitioners. The profession countered that to make the reputations of trained professionals known, they could be licensed. Licensing would not carry rights or privileges but would guarantee that certain examinations had been passed. As a concession to the liberals, the profession admitted that anyone should be allowed to practice medicine.

The idea of a medical register was drawn from a previous private venture by a licentiate of the RCP, a Dr. S. F. Simmons, who had published a medical register in 1779. He had apparently gathered lists of names of practitioners from parts of the country, never claiming to be exhaustive or authoritative, and later published more complete editions in 1780 and 1783.[50] The leaders of the medical profession nearly a century later then converted this type of instrument into an official consumer's guide to the medical profession. Henceforth, only recipients of licenses from professional examining bodies would be registered in the *Medical Register* of the General Medical Council created by the Medical Act of 1858. The state's function evidently would be to guarantee the quality of medical registration. Consumers in the market would be expected to evaluate the performance of medical practitioners, the information in the *Medical Register* forming one part of their judgment of the practitioner. The GMC had no jurisdiction over the quality of practice, only over the quality of education and the maintenance of "profes-

[50] Clark, *op. cit.* (n. 4, above), p. 602.

sional" conduct. The idea of both ethics and "professional" conduct as objects of state responsibility and supervision had been borrowed from the traditions of the RCP; the apothecaries had had no such tradition. Unprofessional conduct did not include mistakes or incompetence short of gross malpractice and gross incompetence.

In short, the state empowered the GMC to enforce legally the traditional internal controls of the medical profession. A registrant found guilty by the GMC of "unprofessional conduct" or convicted of a crime could be stricken from the register. The purpose of the GMC, then, was to be a final authority on the conduct of practitioners. In this way, it helped approach the liberal ideal of selecting practitioners on the basis of their performance. The *Medical Register* reviewed their past performance in training situations; the GMC reviewed their conduct as professionals. Combined, they functioned as an official consumer guide. The penalties for violations support this interpretation of the 1858 Act. Unregistered practice was not criminal. The most serious violation was to procure a place in the register falsely; a less serious offence was to pretend "wilfully and falsely" to be a registered practitioner.[51] In true liberal style, legislation took into account the belief that a rational citizen could investigate for himself whether the practitioner who claimed to be registered was indeed in the register. In fact, using the register to protect prospective patients from unqualified practitioners could be interpreted as a means for fostering the development of greater market consciousness and knowledge. So, by adopting a medical register with legal protection against fraudulent entries, the medical profession not only came to terms with serious libertarian notions of free trade but laid claim to liberal belief in the desirability of improving consumer rationality for a more effective, competitive market.

By changing the nature of medical licensing and permitting free trade, the medical profession also helped reduce strain over another issue. Liberal ideology relied very heavily on the ability of men to be self-interested. It had little room for men who insisted that their ambitions were directed

[51] Burn, *op. cit.*, p. 210.

toward service and not profit. The issue was not whether
or not physicians made profit; that would have been perfectly
agreeable to the liberals. The question was how to overcome
the contradiction between the virtue of a service orientation
and the virtue of a profit orientation. The liberals could not
logically admit that it was morally good in some circumstances to transcend the profit motive, but when the medical
profession adopted the new system of licensing, they did not
have to. According to liberal thought, a professional could
not long escape self-interest, for he would go out of business.
Doctors who could furnish good service to patients would
stay in business; the bad ones would fail. Liberals probably
did not take very seriously those doctors who claimed special
professional authority to determine the true interests of
patients. Liberal logic suggests that doctors are in any event
strongly constrained to demonstrate proof of service in terms
recognizable to the patient in order to maintain authority.
Moreover, if promising to put professional considerations
ahead of profit considerations were found to draw more
patients, then it would be in the self-interest of doctors to
deny their own self-interestedness. As long as society permitted free trade in medicine, the liberals did not care what
the medical profession claimed.

Obviously, state participation in medical affairs was more
difficult to justify to the liberals in view of the laissez faire
components of bourgeois thought. The profession could not
argue that it was pursuing liberal goals but had to demonstrate that at least it was not violating them. Consequently,
the profession took advantage of certain loopholes in liberal
thought to justify less than strict laissez faire attitudes. It
did so with three principles: the state may do what it pleases
so long as free trade is not prevented, the state should act
to maximize individual competition, and the state should
help others to help themselves. The principle of circumscribed state freedom is really a qualification of laissez faire
beliefs by taking the libertarian position. The use of state
action to maximize competition is implicit in pure liberalism.
The doctrine of helping the dependent become independent
is also pure liberalism.

The principle of circumscribed state freedom made possible a number of features of the 1858 Act. The GMC with its *Medical Register* and regulation of licensing, the profession's monopolization of state employment, and the profession's appropriation of suing for fees are all instances of laws which restrain only the state. While laws might not be made to deny Englishmen their liberty, the state could impose any conditions upon itself that it wished. Free trade for others would not be forbidden.

State participation was used to maximize competition by regulating the standards of the licensing corporations by the GMC. Such commentators as Huxley believed that competition among licensing bodies for applicants had led to an apparent decline in the standards of all the bodies. In this case, state intervention could be argued necessary to select socially beneficial types of competition—to reduce competition among licensing bodies but increase it among examinees and teaching institutions. That it would decrease competition among license holders because of the homogenizing effects of more uniform standards was apparently not as important a consideration as making examinations more stringent.

Finally, state intervention was justified by the desirability of making the dependent independent. The task was made easier by the growing sophistication of liberal thought on the problem of social responsibility for the helpless. The liberal mind, insofar as it can be reconstructed, despised weakness, not surprisingly since the rising entrepreneurial class rested its claims to legitimate success on individual strength and ability of its members. The poor in particular were despised for alleged laziness and other imputed moral weaknesses. In an attempt to upgrade the "moral fiber" of the nation, the liberals refused to remove incentives for work. The fear of an uncomfortable life or death by starvation was believed to instill discipline in the lazy poor. The poorhouse system was constructed as an alternative to nonsurvival, but it stigmatized and degraded those placed in it.[52] The

[52] *Ibid.*, ch. 3, pp. 92-129.

role of medical services in this context presented problems for the liberals. Was the helplessness of illness a moral weakness, i.e., one that could be remedied by rational effort?

The Medical Act of 1858 had been passed one year before the publication of Darwin's *Origin of Species*. Later generations might regard the helplessness of the sick as a part of the conflict of nature which eliminates the weak in favor of the fittest, but the generation during which the medical ideology was developed still believed in saving the weak by helping them to help themselves. Part of the problem could be resolved by the principle of encouraging people to make plans for medical care for themselves in advance of trouble. Still, the problem of the relationship of the entrepreneurial elite to illness remained. Was a successful man fallen ill to be considered morally weak? The problem was confronted indirectly at the same time as the passage of the Medical Act in a separate piece of legislation:

> Whatever mid-Victorian England was, it was not a country peopled by doctrinaire lunatics so devoted to laissez-faire that they insisted a free market in arsenic, cheerfully accepted the spread of smallpox and cholera and allowed the victims so produced to be buried at random. The usual, nostalgic ineffective grumbling greeted the Bill of 1860 which became the Act for Preventing the Adulteration of Articles of Food and Drink (23 and 24 Vict, c.84) a somewhat belated outcome of the investigations of the Select Committee of 1856 which had reported that adulteration was habitually practised wherever possible.[53]

Government machinery was set up to analyze the quality of food and drink, upon request and payment of a fee by consumers. But the interesting aspect of this legislation was not so much its deviation from doctrinaire laissez faire as the means used to legitimize it:

> On this, Ayrton (scarcely to be counted among collectivists) asked why tradesmen should not be liable to

[53] *Ibid.*, p. 158.

penalties for cheating poor people and another member,
Wise, said that the poor man had enough to do in earning
his bread without having to analyse it.[54]

This legislation had clearly been passed for the poor. It
might be construed as paternalistic protection of the poor
by the state, but such an interpretation overlooks the ambiguities of the entrepreneurial moral mission. Doctrinaire
laissez faire could fall back on the need for the consumer
to develop market rationality in all purchases as part of
instillation of discipline into the poor. But a laissez faire
philosopher could argue that the development of rationality
and discipline has prerequisites. The entrepreneur's theory
of success was based on the efficacy of hard work; the moral
virtues he should encourage, then, should be those of hard
work. The liberal recognized of course the disadvantageous
position of the poor and the opportunities for exploitation
of their weakness. In most matters the pain of exploitation
would have been morally acceptable as a spur to self-im-
provement. But what if the exploitation killed the naive?
The fear of death could be argued to be an incentive for
self-change, but as the experience of the Poor Law had
suggested, thoughtful liberals were willing to push the morally weak only to the brink, not over it.

There was a place, then, in the liberal mind for extending
protective measures for the poor in medical matters; their
helplessness had to be taken into account in their moral
development. The entrepreneurial class, then, evaded the
problem of its own relative helplessness by protecting the
helpless poor through legislation. The ethical choice was
between creating a jungle or a society of self-reliant, rational
men. Social Darwinism later entertained the former idea,
but the English liberal reformer was able to appeal for
benefits for the sake of others which he could also enjoy
and still protect his own interests without having to confess
weakness. In short, medical licensing appeared as a compensatory device for differences among men in the capacity to
judge the quality of medical practitioners, manifestly intended for those with little knowledge of the reputations of

[54] *Ibid.*

practitioner but useful even for the entrepreneurial elite.

The medical profession's argument in behalf of its own collective interests and existence, then, had shifted function. The claim that the profession was a special case among social institutions was no longer put forward to justify a legal monopoly as much as to justify the new governmental commendatory devices. Tradesmen, craftsmen, and workers did not usually receive licenses from their own guilds as "qualified" representatives. Clearly, the use of licensing gave profession-approved practitioners a privileged position in the market, and this privilege required legitimation. In the process, many in the medical profession changed their minds about the inviolability of professional authority vis-à-vis the government. Though the *Lancet,* the literary arm of the radical medical reformer Thomas Wakely, had declared that Sir James Graham's bill of 1844, which closely resembled the final Medical Act of 1858, would "subject the medical government of this country by means of such [a council], to the control of a minister of the Crown, and the independence of the profession [would be] gone forever,"[55] support and recognition by the state were the established profession's best friend.

Much of the opposition from general practitioners and apothecaries, it would seem, originated from Graham's recognition of the legitimacy of the professional licensing corporations in the bill. The old status struggles between the lower and the higher branches of the profession had been the mitigating factor in the attempt to legislate medical reform. What the reformers had wanted, but did not get, was the elimination of status distinctions by uniform licensing and uniform professional standing; the Graham bill, even when it offered to create a Royal College of General Practitioners, was the government's promise to maintain the status privileges of the separate corporations. Apparently, then, the history of this period was the history of the ideological reformation of the profession to preserve privileges both internally and with respect to larger society in the face of

[55] Arvel B. Erickson, *The Public Career of Sir James Graham* (Oxford: Basil Blackwell; Cleveland: The Press of Western Reserve University, 1952), pp. 247-248.

the levelling forces of liberalism and egalitarianism. With the aid of a few institutional changes and ideological concessions to opponents, the medical profession not only preserved its interest position but possibly improved it.

In summary, the clash between the liberals and the medical profession was resolved in 1858 by the Medical Act, which provided for a number of institutional changes not strictly in keeping with the profession's traditional monopolization strategy of legally privileged restriction and professional autonomy. A new monopolization strategy was apparently constructed, using state administrative devices to give the profession a number of competitive advantages in the market as well as to stabilize the profession's internal institutional arrangements. The new strategy disarmed the attacks of the liberals not only by claiming exemption from liberal theory (through ideological appeals to the liberals), but also by finding loopholes in liberal theory and constructing institutions to fit through those loopholes.

The new monopolization strategy

Having discussed the construction of new institutions and ideologies which led to a new monopolization strategy for the English medical profession, I will now investigate how these institutions have been used to push the collective interests of the medical profession. I will also address the problem of the sense in which the strategy was monopolistic if it had abandoned legal restriction on medical practice.

The question of how the new strategy has been monopolistic is the easier of the two to answer. Though the medical profession after 1858 was not a legally restrictive group, it still had legal privileges. Official recognition in the *Medical Register* gave licensed practitioners a competitive advantage in the open market, but there is a more important respect in which, the new strategy was monopolistic. Since the Medical Act permitted the state to employ only registered medical practitioners, the medical profession had won a legal monopoly on state consumption of medical services. This arrangement tended to do away with the problem of legal enforcement of legal privileges, for the state did not have to support this type of monopolization by apprehending, prosecuting, convicting, and punishing illegal practitioners— an inefficient and limited means at best for eliminating external competitors. But the medical profession subsequently had to face the problem of applying this limited monopolization in behalf of the group's interests.

The answer in retrospect seems simple enough: maximize income from the state by converting medical practitioners into state employees and encouraging patients to use state-employed doctors. Though many in the medical profession resisted this line of development for a variety of reasons, the remarkable thing is that the history of medical organization in England during the twentieth century followed it to a surprisingly close degree. The National Health Insurance Act of 1912 and the National Health Service Act of 1946 both illustrate how the new strategy was implemented. The National Health Insurance plan (NHI) provided for free medical care for workers who voluntarily subscribed to the plan. Patients signed up on a panel to receive care from a doctor of their choice, who was then paid from a central fund according to the number of patients on the panel (capitation fees). The National Health Service (NHS) extended this type of plan to cover all interested patients who wished to subscribe to the service. With certain minor exceptions, the NHS provided comprehensive services free upon demand. NHS doctors were paid either by the NHI system of capitation fees, if they were general practitioners, or by salary, if they were hospital-based consultants.[56] These governmentally financed service plans encouraged patients to use state-employed doctors, i.e., those with licenses, by making available free services, a powerful competitive device within the open market.

Interestingly enough, even this economic inducement has not been sufficient to bring about complete patient use of state services; even though 100 percent of licensed practitioners work for the NHS, some patients still choose non-

[56] Rosemary Stevens, *Medical Practice in Modern England: The Impact of Specialization and State Medicine* (New Haven and London: Yale University Press, 1966), pp. 36-37, 91-92.

NHS practitioners or see NHS practitioners on a private, fee-for-service basis for noneconomic reassons.[57] Yet the use of state employment and financing to induce patients to use "free" NHS practitioners represents the ultimate logical conclusion of the new monopolization strategy.

Because the profession's chief source of income has shifted to the state under the new monopolization strategy, the old devices for maximizing income have become inadequate. The sliding scale and uniform fees may have worked sufficiently well when patients were atomized employers of the doctor, but the state is in a much less vulnerable position than the patient. How, then, has the medical profession in England attempted to maximize the profession's total income?

Essentially, the medical profession must request income increases from the government, and it has developed two general tactics to win these. The general practitioners have tended to use collective-bargaining tactics, while the elitist groups within the profession—such as the RCP—have tended to use more subtle means.

The first type of tactics has been the familiar pressure group politics of the British Medical Association (BMA), whose actions and relationship to the government are, as will be seen, comparable to some of those of the American Medical Association in the United States. The BMA arose to defend the general practitioner's interests, even though its membership also included consultants. Rosemary Stevens has called the Medical Act of 1858 the best friend of the general practitioners because it created one profession, and indeed the Act provided them with a monopolization of state employment which later economically supported them.[58] Nonetheless, the government has repeatedly treated the general practitioners as stepchildren of the profession. Beforehand, they had certainly never shared in the privileges or prestige of the Royal Colleges. The 1858 Act still distinguished them from the physicians and surgeons as before. The role of the government with respect to the general practitioners and their apothecary ancestors had been to

[57] *Ibid.*, p. 206.
[58] *Ibid.*, p. 24.

outlaw their practice, then to restrict it to specific geographical areas and prevent them from enjoying equal prestige with the Colleges. This sort of treatment seemingly made the general practitioners hostile toward the government; despite concessions, the government continually frustrated many general-practitioner interests. This hostility led to an antigovernmental bias which contributed to the development of general-practitioner bargaining with the government to secure their interests.

A confrontational approach to profession-state relations has not been universal throughout the organized English medical profession. The Royal Colleges have developed close ties with the ruling Establishment and informal connections with influential persons so that the interests of these groups could be furthered through direct requests. From the time of Henry VIII, when the RCP could legitimately request help on the basis of its liturgical relationship to the Crown, until the present National Health Service, the Royal Colleges have defined the profession-state relationship as cordial and cooperative. They have used techniques of friendly informal persuasion behind the scenes, not demands or threats of withdrawal of efficiency. Positive evidence for such understandings is of course scarce because of their nonpublic, hence invisible, nature. Perhaps the best example of the difference is provided in this passage from Stevens concerning a meeting during the summer of 1946, two years before the NHS opened its doors:

Representing the GP's, the association [the BMA] held bitter protest meetings against certain provisions in the Bill. Its mood of calm reasonableness evaporated, and it seemed to have forgotten its earlier dicta on the influence of the profession in the National Health Insurance scheme. Meanwhile the Royal Colleges gave impressive and apparently cordial dinners for members of the government. Their aristocratic lineage held firm; at times their links with the royal family appeared stronger than those with their brothers in general practice. The Princess Royal visited the Royal College of Surgeons,

of which she was an honorary Fellow, to look at their
plans for rebuilding, in the month in which the Bill was
laid before Parliament, and again later to pay tribute
to a survey of anesthesiology before the Bill was enacted.
While it was in committee stage and general practitioners' feelings were at their height, the Queen gra-
ciously accepted the office of Patron of the Royal College
of Obstetricians and Gynaecologists. That same month
(June 1946) the Labour Prime Minister, a Hunterian
trustee, attended a dinner at the Royal College of
Surgeons. Other examples can be enumerated of the
interplay of the Royal Colleges with the social "establishment" of England. "The college spirit in medicine,"
said Eardley Holland, President of the Royal College
of Obstetricians and Gynaecologists [founded in 1929]
at a dinner at that college in September 1946, "is pre-
cious, is unique, and is peculiarly British, and its flame
must never die down." The power of the Colleges, the
President emphasized, have depended not on privileges
but on cultural and even spiritual qualities; and it was
essential that they should achieve unity and harmony.
He might have been addressing a group of British subal-
terns in the outposts of Empire, or the assembled body
of an English public school. Beside this suave rhetoric,
the activities of the BMA appeared rough and naive.[59]

Whenever possible, the medical profession has used state
administrative structures to further its collective interests.
Several areas have already been mentioned in which the state
has assumed authority in medical affairs; but even while
the state has assumed the formal authority to decide such
matters as eligibility for state employment, exclusion from
the *Medical Register,* and the adequacy of licensing examinations, the professional bodies have exercised great influence on the decisions of the state, particularly of the General
Medical Council and the Ministry of Health. Partly this is
because professionals dominate certain structures such as
the GMC by legal majority representation but also because

[59] *Ibid.*, pp. 77-78.

Ministers of Health typically lack both expertise and incentive to oppose the organized professional bodies. The National Health Service as part of the welfare state is very much a politicized service, and the Minister of Health's primary responsibility is to see that it stays in operation with a modicum of efficiency and effectiveness. Part of his job, necessarily, is to satisfy enough of practitioner interests to maintain productivity at an adequate level. Generally, he can do so by yielding to professional preferences.

Yet in some areas, such as income for state-employed practitioners, the influence of the professional bodies is relatively more constrained. Disputes over governmental payments have been numerous since 1948 and on several occasions have threatened to close down the NHS. Yet, interestingly enough, they have not done so. Although the Ministry of Health has been willing to maintain relatively high practitioner income levels for the sake of winning professional cooperation with the NHS, a number of contradictions in the system have acted as constraints. Initially, practitioner incomes were to have been set at the level of private practice, but the system's built-in tendency to eliminate private practice through price competition has made private-practice incomes an unsuitable and arbitrary standard. Also, for a variety of reasons, the Ministry of Health has refused to link doctors' income to an abstract principle such as the rising cost of living or other measures of general economic development.[60] Instead, the Ministry has offered incomes which provide the minimum personnel necessary to run the Service. Essentially, the Ministry has tried to minimize costs while maximizing services. What practitioners in the NHS are paid, therefore, is heavily determined by the services the Ministry is prepared to buy. What the Ministry can buy is in turn heavily determined by Parliamentary budgetary limitations. The NHS has an important built-in contradiction: the government is ideologically committed to provide comprehensive services, but services are potentially infinite and the government has limited resources. Essentially, the government must decide priorities among medical

[60] *Ibid.*, p. 133.

services and priorities relative to other national objectives.

An abstractly conceived rationality of professional action calls for the all-out commitment of resources for medical services regardless of other considerations. If the profession can influence the government to allocate large amounts for medical services, it may well serve its collective interests as well as service interests. In this respect, the arguments between the organized British profession and the state over professional incomes and budgets do not at all necessarily indicate loss of professional domination. The English public has invested progressively less for medical services in the open market than in central planning. As the allocation of national resources comes under the authority of a central planning system, the profession's opportunities for achieving larger allocations become greater, for the revenue base increases through taxation and other funding devices. From this perspective, economic conflict between government and state has not been due so much to governmental stinginess as to the new opportunities for satisfying the profession's interests through the introduction of central planning and the creation of new sources for income.

The history of the British medical profession suggests that the profession has been far more successful influencing the opinion of the government than of the public at large; concomitantly, the profession has had to please the government much more than previously. The current political problem of the profession no longer seems to be one of justifying privileges but of winning greater allocations by convincing th government of the importance of more medical services and more complicated medical services.[61] Since at least 1946 under the NHS, the British government has been morally committed to providing for all medical needs through the established profession. It has also been acutely aware that economic scarcities make strict fulfillment of this commitment impossible. Out of this disparity comes the profession's new domination problem: to influence favorably where the government will draw the line for permissible services.

[61] John Lister, "By the London Post," *New England Journal of Medicine* 285 (25 November 1971), pp. 1247-1249.

The development of national health care delivery systems in England has not been inconsistent with the interests of the medical profession but even seems to be a logical conclusion of the monopolization strategy formed by the awarding of new privileges in 1858. Although probably not anticipated but rather capitalized upon, the NHI and the NHS have not so much altered the character of the profession's organization as they have developed it in a monopolistic direction, taking advantage of the profession's monopolization of state employment. While everyday practice may or may not be different under these systems, they have not changed the fundamental strategy by which the profession has tended to pursue its interests since the mid-nineteenth century. The profession has simply developed more effective tactics and administrative relationships to make use of the increased potential for interest satisfaction in its relationship to the state. In retrospect, the liberal threat to the existence of the medical profession ironically resulted in institutional changes which, though unanticipated, improved the interest position of the profession once the state began to play a significant role in distributing services to the nation.

Recapitulation

This chapter has followed how the modern concept of the medical profession as an autonomous legally privileged group of practitioners arose, despite the constraints of the traditional system of medieval guilds, and has traced the profession from its origins in the Royal College of Physicians, first a royally privileged group and then a legislatively privileged group, as it early acquired the authority to eliminate external competition. Subsequent to its rise, the profession underwent two phases of apparent demonopolization. First, the concept of the profession was extended beyond the boundaries of the RCP to include a number of other licensed groups of practitioners, apparently an example of failing to eliminate certain external competitors and so admitting them into the legally privileged group. Later, the medical profession lost its status as a legal monopoly in the open market, seemingly inviting unlicensed practitioners to compete with licensed practitioners. These apparent examples of demonopolization, however, on closer examination were not compromises of the monopolization interests of the profession but instead shifts in monopolization strategy in response to changing political conditions.

The RCP's original monopolization rights were probably directed at the market of the royal court, even though they formally provided for the entire English market for medical services. Other groups of practitioners acquired legal privileges only on the condition that the RCP's original monopolization of the court and prominent people not be broken. As such, extension of legal privileges to other practitioner groups helped clarify monopolization rights for each group, more or less dividing the national service market into separate domains. Limited legal privileges had been given to these groups to induce them to refrain from illegal competition, which could otherwise not be curtailed on account of poor enforcement and the relatively great net shortage of licensed physicians.

Opening up the right to practice medicine to the public also did not constitute true demonopolization. In the face of powerful opposition from liberal political groups and ideologies, the medical profession changed its institutional relationships to the state, relying on the state less to enforce restrictions on practice and more to augment the profession's prestige and market value, thereby defusing liberal objections to a considerable extent. These institutional changes set the stage for the twentieth century, during which the profession's monopolization of state employment has diminished external competition by creating medical service plans financed by the state to offer services free at the point of delivery—the ultimate in price competition in the open market.

It is now possible to better clarify the role of the concept of the legally privileged group in Weber's theory of monopolization. Monopolistic authority, even legal authority, in the open market need not result in authoritative, empirical domination of the market. This is because restrictive privileges are effective only insofar as they are enforced, and enforcement is evidently often problematic. Weber's concept of legal privileges, however, need not narrowly consider only

formal grants of monopoly. Other types of legal privileges
can result in remarkably effective de facto monopolization.
Legally privileged access to state employment, for instance,
poses few problems of enforcement yet provides monopolization benefits in two senses: effective price competition
through free state distribution of services, and a potentially
greater source of income for the profession. Even so, a
potentially greater income may not be realized for political
reasons, since the state must be persuaded to allocate income
favorably for medical services, and allocations are subject
to a variety of considerations. Hence, because the consequences of legal privileges for an interest group's monopolization, particularly with respect to eliminating external
competition, depend on political conditions, the type of
privileges that the group may find most to its advantage
varies according to circumstance. As will now be shown, the
types of legal privileges acquired by the medical profession
in the United States have differed from those of the contemporary English profession, for the most part because of
different political and legal conditions.

CHAPTER FIVE

The American Medical Profession:
Licensure and Monopolization

In the previous chapter about the medical profession in
England, the paradox of the monopolistic consequences of
apparent demonopolization was dealt with by examining the
profession's organizational strategy within its changing context. It seemed particularly enlightening the way restrictive
legal privileges, reduced from the sphere of the market to
state employment, had been in time turned to competitive
advantage for the profession. In this chapter on the American
medical profession, I shall similarly seek instances of apparent demonopolization in order to explore heuristically their
actual monopolistic consequences within the profession's
political setting. My purpose is to go beyond the already
stated model of monopolization to discover how the medical
profession has been institutionalized as a profession in
America and so contribute to a more comprehensive monopolization model. I shall accept arguments in the literature
that assert that the American medical profession has tended
to be monopolistic, for the evidence in this chapter is not
intended to prove the thesis that the profession has been
monopolistic—that I concede for the purposes of theory-
building. I want to distinguish the respects in which the
profession has been monopolistic, and the reasons it has been
monopolistic in the ways it has, in order to increase understanding of monopolization.

In this chapter on American licensure, licensing will be used as in the English chapter: to investigate the different roles it has played in the profession's monopolization strategies. As before, the monopolization strategies of the American medical profession will be investigated. As in the English chapter, explanations for changes of strategy will be sought in the profession's political context.

The monopolization strategy of the Royal College of Physicians

Unlike the English profession, American practitioners could borrow an organizational model: the English RCP. The study of the American profession, therefore, begins with the colonial period to adequately investigate the relationship of American practitioners to the RCP's type of monopolization strategy under the conditions present in American political institutions. The Royal College of Physicians did not extend professional status to the surgeons until the late part of the eighteenth century or to the apothecaries until the early part of the nineteenth century. Before the English tripartite profession came into being, the American Revolution had already occurred. The idea of the profession in America, then, remained the model of the RCP, and as shall be seen, some American doctors attempted to emulate it.

The adoption of the RCP's model of the profession and its monopolization strategy did not mean that American doctors attempted to copy the RCP's structure in every detail. One must consider it in the context of the problem of the ways in which an interest group might maximize the processes mentioned in the theory of monopolization. Essentially, the RCP model as a logically coherent type suggests that monopolization is most effective through maximization of the interest group's control in a number of spheres. The model calls for the formation of a group in which membership can be held, control over the structure of that group (its boundaries, size, and composition), and control over the technical, social, and economic conduct of its members. The group directly exerts control over group structure and member conduct through the group's own machinery (the means of control) and places control over the means of group enforcement in the hands of the group's leadership. The group's leadership also makes policies to determine rationally and specifically the structure and conduct of the group. In all these matters, directness of control is important to help implement the policies of the group in an exact manner.

As applied to the medical profession, this model is consistent with the RCP's status as a licensing corporation, using medical licensing as a restrictive mechanism administered by a practitioner-dominated organization, issuing licenses at the group's discretion, and punishing violators. Historically, the RCP model represents practitioner domination of practitioner activities in all areas, using a self-regulating group structure, fraternalistic members bound together by status conventions, but employing other sanctions to control its membership. It is distinguished from systems of practitioners dominated by laymen or academics or from systems where control of group structure and membership conduct is exercised through institutional machinery outside the group. In these respects, it overlaps with the guild as a self-regulating fraternal consociation, although as I argued in the preceding chapter, its political status has differed from that of the guild.

Lamentably, one does not find sociologists who have analyzed the American medical profession as an example of practitioner-dominated monopolization. The last sociological work to take the monopolistic nature of the professions seriously, Carr-Saunder's *The Professions,* studied only British professions.[1] For interpretations in terms of monopolization, one must turn to journalists, historians, economists, lawyers, and even certain physicians. An excellent study of the American Medical Association as a monopoly, for example, was presented by the editors of the 1954 *Yale Law Journal.*[2] Perhaps the best analytical statement on the monopolistic nature of the American medical profession is

---

[1] A. M. Carr-Saunders, and P. A. Wilson, *The Professions* (Oxford: The Clarendon Press, 1933), pp. 352-365.

[2] David R. Hyde and Staff, "The American Medical Association: Power, Purpose, and Politics in Organized Medicine," *Yale Law Journal* 63 (May 1954), pp. 938-1022.

an essay by the political economist Milton Friedman, whose own philosophical views are similar to those of nineteenth-century English liberals. His recommendation that medical licensure should be abolished in favor of medical certification seems unlikely to be heeded and ignores many major public-interest issues in planning medical services, but this does not reduce the clarity of his statement and insights. It is a particularly useful place to begin, since he appreciates the central institutional importance of licensing as a monopolistic device.

Milton Friedman's theory of American professional control mechanisms in medicine

According to Friedman, the American Medical Association is perhaps the strongest trade union in America, and like any trade union, derives its power from its ability to restrict the number of those who engage in an occupation. The American Medical Association restricts admission to the profession by two major mechanisms: restriction of admission to medical schools and restriction of the legal right to practice by licensing requirements. These two mechanisms tend to be linked; in almost every state, graduation from a medical school approved by the Council on Medical Education and Hospitals of the American Medical Association is a prerequisite for licensing. Moreover, the members of licensing commissions are virtually always physicians. While licensing boards have restricted membership by denying licenses to already trained foreign physicians on the basis of citizenship and language requirements, control of admissions to medical school is generally more important than over licensing boards. This is because students who have already made an investment in their career educations are likely to persist in trying to pass licensing examinations until they are successful. Control over medical school admissions, therefore, is more restrictive because it simply turns down many applicants and, more subtly, discourages many potential applicants from even trying. The means of control are the high standards and requirements necessary for admission and the strong influence of the Committee on Medical

Education of the American Medical Association on medical school admissions committees: "For example, in the 1930's, during the depression, the Council on Medical Education and Hospitals wrote a letter to the various medical schools saying the medical schools were admitting more students than could be given the proper kind of training. In the next year or two, every school reduced the number it was admitting, giving very strong presumptive evidence that the recommendation had some effect."[3] Compliance with such requests from the American Medical Association is obtained through the authority of the American Medical Association to designate approved and unapproved medical schools.

Control by the AMA over the conduct of practitioners is attained through a parallel mechanism: the approval of hospitals. Hospitals, for their part, exert control over physicians by providing staff (admitting) privileges. Approval is important to hospitals, since they require inexpensive interns and residents to operate at minimal expense, and internships are acceptable to licensing boards only when taken at approved hospitals. This control has been used to regulate the economic and social conduct of physicians, by withdrawing staff privileges from physicians who participate in AMA—disapproved health plans, particularly prepaid group practice, apparently to eliminate the possibility of engaging in discriminatory pricing.

Friedman then goes on to the problem of the public-interest consequences of licensure, which are somewhat incidental to this chapter, and argues that medical licensing has violated the public interest by rendering standards of practice (not education) low. It reduces the number of physicians, the number of hours available for physicians to perform more rather than fewer less important tasks, and the incentive for research and development (by limiting research for the main part to practitioners or licensed potential practitioners). It also discourages physicians from testifying in malpractice suits in behalf of plaintiffs and from experimenting with health care delivery systems. Friedman's solu-

---

[3] Milton Friedman, *Capitalism and Freedom* (Chicago: University of Chicago Press, 1962), p. 150.

tion is to remove licensing requirements and leave the development of collectivized systems of health care delivery up to the market. He does not propose that individual practice simply be left open to anyone; he wants to see the system of practitioner domination become sufficiently open to permit the development of "department stores of medicine," in which the quality of professional practice would be more visible and in which practitioners could exert more rational control over one another's technical performance. He also is willing to permit individual practitioners, however, on the basis of a philosophical commitment to consumer sovereignty and market diversity.[4]

Critique of Friedman

Friedman's comments are, by and large, accurate and penetrating. If anything, they underestimate the extensiveness of control of this system. The state medical licensing boards are composed usually of representatives of state medical societies, either appointed or nominated by state medical societies. Often, these are former officers of medical societies.[5] Even more important than board composition may be the medical practice acts which set requirements for medical education.[6] These acts tend to reduce admissions by setting spiraling standards for medical schools, making education long, expensive, and difficult for schools to keep pace with. Providing sufficient hospital and instructor contacts for a wide variety of medical subjects for all students is one example of how this process works. The capacity of the medical schools to keep pace with inflating standards has also been curtailed in the twentieth century by the AMA's consistent policy of preventing governmental financing or subsidies for medical education.[7] And even with the introduction of some measure of federal financing of medical

---

[4] *Ibid.*, pp. 149-160.

[5] Robert C. Derbyshire, *Medical Licensure and Discipline in the United States* (Baltimore and London: Johns Hopkins Press, 1969), pp. 33-34.

[6] *Ibid.*, pp. 13-30.

[7] Elton Rayack, *Professional Power and American Medicine: The Economics of the American Medical Association* (Cleveland and New York: The World Publishing Company, 1967), pp. 79-94.

[8] Anne R. Somers, *Hospital Regulation: The Dilemma of Public Policy* (Princeton, New Jersey: Princeton University, 1969), p. 23.

schools, the schools have found it in their interest to hold admissions levels low in order to augment their bargaining position with the government over income and other matters. The outcome is that even though the AMA has reversed its traditional policy of restriction of numbers of physicians and has called for expansion since 1965, the number of new medical schools built and additional medical students graduated has been minimal.

With respect to hospitals, too, Friedman appears to be limited in comprehensiveness. Until 1963, approved hospitals did not extend staff privileges to practitioners who were not members of medical societies, because of pressures from the organized profession. Court decisions, however, have prohibited this practice.[8] This former interlocking domination of medical society and hospital contributed to the meaningfulness of the sanction of expulsion from medical societies, such as for unethical practice in the form of participating in disapproved health plans. Since the judicial breaking of this connection, membership in the AMA and medical societies has declined,[9] in part because it is no longer essential for practice in community hospitals. Yet another omission by Friedman is the power of licensing boards dominated by medical societies to revoke licenses for a variety of reasons, among them, unprofessional conduct, a term undefined by law. Even though there is legal recourse to revocation through the courts, the device still has considerable value as a control mechanism.[10]

A more important shortcoming of Friedman's work is that it offers no explanation for why the network of controls over

[9] The percentage of the medical profession who hold membership in the AMA has declined over the past decade. The following figures are based on computerized membership rolls, which were not available prior to 1963:

1963	73.2%	1968	68.5%
1964	72.5%	1969	67.7%
1965	72.3%	1970	65.6%
1966	71.7%	1971	60.6%
1967	69.9%		

"It should be pointed out that, over the years, of those office based physicians, approximately 80-85% have availed themselves of an AMA membership. The overall proportion of AMA members to the entire medical profession is obviously smaller than that because of the physicians involved in teaching, government and research." No detailed substantiation of this claim is provided, however, in this personal communication (letter) by Timothy B. Norbeck, assistant director, Department of Specialty Society Services, American Medical Association, 7 June 1972.

[10] Derbyshire, *op. cit.*, pp. 85-86.

practitioners is diffuse. He is acutely aware of how much entry into the profession is restricted and how effectively control over practitioners' conduct can be constructed, yet misses the point that control is indirectly applied by the AMA. While these control methods may be relatively effective means for monopolization, remarkably they have been applied by nonpractitioner-dominated health-related institutions, such as state licensing boards, medical schools, and hospitals. That is, why is control not applied directly through the system of organized medical societies and the AMA, particularly since medical professional ideologies state that regulation and control of practitioners should rest in the hands of practitioners? Control seemingly does rest in the hands of the organized profession ultimately, but there is an element of indirectness which requires explanation.

Another area for investigation which Friedman does not adequately address is the role of the AMA in medical control. His writings and also the classic article on the AMA in the *Yale Law Journal* imply that an oligarchical AMA controls physicians throughout the nation through its organizational arms, the state and local medical societies. According to this view, the core of organized medicine's domination rests in the hands of the AMA, and state and local societies are merely subordinate puppets to take care of the details of dominating hospitals, medical schools, and licensing boards on a local level. While this model is not inherently illogical, it is not consistent with the degree of decentralization in the system. The formation of the AMA preceded the formation of state licensing boards. Was there, then, any monopolistic significance in the AMA's creating decentralized state rather than federal licensing boards? Since the AMA's committees evaluate medical schools and hospitals for approval and accreditation, why was there interposed the complex and relatively more indirect means of local medical society control? In short, if the AMA has been the key point of control of practitioners, why has it employed indirect and decentralized control mechanisms?

Deviations from the RCP's monopolization strategy

As Friedman's essay implicitly suggests, the contemporary American medical profession does not conform to the RCP's model of monopolization. Although it appears that the medical societies heavily influenced group structure, the means of control are indirect through nonpractitioner institutions, and membership size is determined by setting minimal requirements (i.e., obstacles to entry) instead of maximum membership numbers. There is direct control over member conduct in the sense that at least one group institutional means of control exists: expulsion from medical society membership. Because of the indirectness of practitioner control by state licensing boards, however, nonmembership in medical societies does not preclude the right to practice, that is, to membership in the legal medical profession. This indirectness of control tends to weaken the value of medical society membership as a sanction.

An examination of the historical literature of the American medical profession suggests other types of deviations of major significance. The examples of the contemporary American use of indirect means of practitioner-group domination contrast with past instances of virtually no practitioner domination of existing control institutions. Following a petition from the New Jersey Medical Society to the provincial legislature requesting the establishment of a system of medical practice legislation, the legislature passed a statute in 1772 providing for licensing of practitioners through the Supreme Court and requesting that the advice of any persons whom the court saw fit be drawn upon. This case will be more thoroughly discussed in another context, below. For now, it is important to illustrate how legal means could restrict the supply of practitioners in the market without direct or indirect control by practitioners. Even though an interest group, the New Jersey Medical Society, had been formed, licensing and

[11] George Rosen, "Fee and Fee Bills: Some Economic Aspects of Medical Practice in Nineteenth Century America," *Bulletin of the History of Medicine* Supplement 6 (1946), pp. 1-91.

therefore restriction of membership were not the privileged domain of the group. Instead, judicial licensing created an independently defined group of practitioners, outside the control of the interest group. Obviously, such a system limits the potential of the interest group to control the larger group's structure and membership conduct. In terms of monopolization, this case illustrates how a mere restriction of supply by licensing constitutes monopolization only in a limited and weak sense in the absence of interest-group control.

To illustrate how ineffective control of physicians' conduct might be in the absence of interest-group control, there is the example of the use of fee bills or tables of fees issued by medical societies during the nineteenth century[11] at a time when entry into practice could be legally achieved through either medical society licensing or medical school diplomas, and later in the century, when entry was open to all. In hopes of establishing a system of traditional fees, sets of minimum fees for procedures were issued. In light of an understanding of monopolization strategies, these attempts were predictably liable to failure because of the absence of comprehensive interest-group control of physicians' economic conduct. The result was that "ethical" medical society members could be readily underbid by non-member practitioners, and adherence to the tables of fees threatened to price medical society members' services out of the market. As a method of fee fixing, as a form of economic conduct, the fee table was bound to fail because of a failure to lay the infrastructure of membership restriction and control of conduct.

From one perspective, these examples of medical society deviations from an ideal model of monopolization strategy might be evidence against monopolistic intent. It might be that institutional devices desired for various reasons, such as reducing conflicts between patients and physicians with respect to issues of fair fees, resembled devices which might be monopolistic in another context, but that this resemblance was only coincidental. A different explanation in the instances of the New Jersey licensing law and medical society fee bills is that the medical societies did not know what they were doing, that they were naive about the political requirements for monopolization. In this case, the question of intent is not of particular explanatory importance. Without an adequate system of practitioner controls by the medical societies, fee bills were likely to fail because of the nature of the operation of the open market, unless the marginal utility of services by medical society members were increased over those of nonmembers, and that was unlikely for a number of historical reasons. Similarly, in the New Jersey case, it was the failure of the medical society to establish strong influence over court licensing machinery and over the provincial legislature which blocked monopolization and disappointed some medical leaders by permitting the licensing of practitioners of whom they disapproved. In these cases, both economic and ideal interests tended to require more sophisticated monopolization, which makes the issue of specific motivation rather irrelevant.

The issue at the heart of these deviations is the degree of separation of interest-group domination from the means of control. To maximize the group's collective interests, the group needs to exercise control, for the willingness of outsiders to protect the interests of the group is uncertain. To see a separation of practitioner domination (as opposed to lay or academic domination) from the means of control, then, is not remarkable. Two problems of explanation arise in view of this deviation from a model monopolization strategy: (1) what political devices can compensate for this separation from the means of control, i.e., overcome it when direct control is not formally permitted? (2) why is there a separation?

Compensation for separation from the means of control

While any interest group should rationally have a representative organization to work for privileges and controls, in the face of separation from the means of control such an ideally rational organization should also establish domination over external institutions exercising direct control over practitioners. In a sense, these political centers for the interest group are more important under conditions of separation, to counteract the tendency of external institutions to act autonomously. If the interest group wins direct control privileges over practitioners, it will not likely have to continue rewinning them as can be the case with indirect control relationships. In the case of the American medical profession, interest-group formation has occurred in the form of the medical societies, and these organizations have borne the brunt of dominating external health institutions.

Domination does not happen merely by fiat; effective means of domination must be created. Under conditions of separation, means of domination over external institutions are necessary to compensate for the separation. These means may be either legal or extralegal. Legal means in the United States are illustrated by the legal right of state medical societies to appoint or nominate members of state medical examination boards. An alternative legal means might be the right to veto appointments, but this means has not been used in medicine so far. Also, state medical-practice laws which set licensing requirements and exert pressure on medical schools are a legal means of domination, even if secured by extralegal means of influence, e.g., lobbying. Other extralegal means include recommendations to medical schools regarding optimal numbers of admissions, recommendations to hospitals concerning staffing privileges, in short, the phenomena which have previously been discussed. To be effective, these means of domination must have accompanying sanctions, such as threats of loss of accreditation or approved status. The use of sanctions by the medical societies has already been discussed above and requires no further comment.

A useful compensatory tactic is the exclusion of laymen from policy-making positions in external institutions. While not always possible, any degree of exclusion makes separation less important, for the interests of the medical societies can be better represented. A mere demand for practitioner leadership in external institution permits practitioners unsympathetic to medical society policies and interests to occupy these positions, but apparently the sanctions exercised by the societies effectively prevent their appointment. The interests of the medical societies are thus represented in two ways: by the harmony of values, interests, and beliefs of appointed medical society members with the medical society, and by a willingness to comply with official and informal recommendations from the medical society.

Independent sources of practitioner economic support also help establish domination over external institutions. For practitioners serving as policy makers in external institutions, this tendency may be expressed as gratuitous service on medical examination committees or planning councils. While a practitioner who serves in this capacity may lose some income, he remains loyal to the medical society. One of the more plausible arguments against participation of physicians in lay-sponsored plans is that economic dependence on laymen may compromise technical judgment. Not far beyond this argument is the more general argument that economic dependence of practitioners tends to lead to loss of practitioner control in all matters. Practitioner domination may, of course, persist even under conditions of economic dependence, but the combination lacks stability. (The organized American profession has tended to be rather purist in its demands for economic independence, seeing virtually any form of economic dependence of practitioners on organized laymen as an actual, and not merely potential, threat to practitioner domination.) This line of reasoning, that medical society representatives should not be subject to the economic power of the institutions they are trying to dominate, seems to be more applicable to those within policy-making positions in those institutions than to participant physicians who provide services, since the former are the main carriers of medical society interests.

These compensations for separation from the means of control, then, are important because they constitute a logical alternative monopolization strategy to the RCP's. By authoritatively dominating external institutions, the medical societies use them for de facto domination of practitioners in a monopolistic direction. In this respect, the distinctiveness of the American medical profession's current monopolization strategy seems to be precisely its use of indirect and diffuse controls.

Toward a historically grounded explanation for separation from controls

Why has the American medical profession adopted an indirect and diffuse type of monopolization strategy? To answer this question, I shall turn in search of structural clues to the history of the American medical profession's attempts at organization. What features of American society and its political and legal structure have led to the medical profession's adopting this alternative monopolization strategy? In the English chapter, I investigated the effects of anti-monopolistic ideologies on the institutions of the English medical profession. In this chapter, I will do the same, recognizing that American antimonopolistic ideologies may be of a different nature than in England. I shall inquire into which American ideologies were antimonopolistic, and the role that they played in the construction of a new type of monopolization strategy for the medical profession. Finally, to add a new type of question that I failed to raise in the English chapter, I shall investigate the political conditions under which antimonopolistic ideologies affect or do not affect the profession's institutionalization.

Since one is not interested in every change that the profession underwent, one can look at the profession in terms of its response to changing structural conditions in American society. Therefore, the history of the organized medical profession will be separated into periods according to changes in corporate law. I have selected corporate law for several reasons. Corporate law has tended to be more uniform both spatially and temporally than professional organization, and has even been national in scope, occasionally taking the form of federal laws. By holding changes in corporate law constant, so to speak, one can then study changes in professional organization. Perhaps a classification system based on shifting patterns of political interests in American politics would ultimately be more satisfactory, but for now, corporate law will have to act as a halfway house between political interests

nings of colonization of the New World and only gradually
and professional organization. By focusing on corporate law,
one can hope to understand a little of both.

The four periods which will be used here include the
following: the prohibition of corporation, special incorporation legislation, general incorporation legislation, and antitrust legislation. There is a certain amount of overlap between
general corporation laws and antitrust legislation, in that
the first provides for the creation of certain types of corporations and the second regulates their conduct and relationships. Yet antitrust legislation has had such a profound
influence on the normative theory of corporate organization
in American society, particularly with respect to permissible
types, that it will be treated as a separate phase.

The prohibition of corporations

Political soil for the creation of a local medical profession
of organized practitioners was very inhospitable at the begin-
became more favorable as political relations with the mother
country changed. Under English common law, the chartering
of corporations by a corporation was illegal.[12] Inasmuch as
colonial settlements were chartered corporations, their administrative machinery was not believed to possess the right
to incorporate local corporations, in this case, medical societies. Even if medical societies had been incorporated, as in
time they were despite common law tradition, they could
have had no licensing privileges because of the preexisting
monopoly on licensing held by the Royal College of Physicians in London. Underlying such constraints was a built-in
ambiguity about the status of the American colonies, an
unanticipated development in administrative law. Were
American settlers still Englishmen? Were they subject to
the same rights and obligations as other Englishmen, despite
the great distance from the home country and difficulties
in enforcing certain regulations over great distances? Did
the jurisdiction of English institutions extend to the colo-

---

[12] Joseph Stancliffe Davis, *Essays in the Earlier History of American Corporations: Eighteenth Century Business Corporations in the United States*, 2 vols. (New
York: Russell & Russell, 1965), vol. I, p. 20.

nies? Was the English government responsible for the welfare of colonial settlers? As long as these questions were answered affirmatively, especially on the American side of the ocean, there was little hope for the development of self-regulating medical institutions in America. There is little evidence of such attempts during early colonial American history, but this may well be because of the discouraging political and legal context instead of mere lack of interest in monopolization.

The earliest medical regulation law in English colonial America both contributed to the discouragement of interest-group formation and yet contained the seeds for their formation. A Virginia law of 1639 apparently threatened medical practitioners with arrest if they charged "excessive fees." Some clues as to the rationale behind this law are suggested by the preamble to the Virginian act of 1646, which essentially reaffirmed the regulatory law of 1639:

> Whereas the 9th act of the assembly held the 21st of October, 1639, consideration being had and taken of the immoderate and excessive rates and prices exacted by practitioners in physic and churyrgery and the complaints made to the then Assembly of the bad consequences thereof. It so happening through the said intollerable exactions that the hearts of divers masters were hardened rather to suffer their servants to perish for want of fitt meanes and applications than by seeking reliefe to fall into the hands of griping and avaricious men.[13]

The reference to the consequences of medical economic conduct for the master-servant relationship suggests that perhaps something more than the welfare sentiments of traditional paternalism was at stake. It does not seem unreasonable to speculate, in light of the financial responsibility of Virginia tobacco plantations to English investors, that maintaining settlement costs at a minimum was a major

[13] Henry Burnell Shafer, *The American Medical Profession, 1783-1850* (New York: AMS Press, 1936), p. 204.

administrative concern of the colonists. There is apparently
some evidence that the English exerted pressure on the
Virginians to return substantial profits,[14] which would have
given the Virginians particular interest in minimizing all
costs, including the costs of maintaining plantation workers
in working condition. It is important to emphasize that the
Virginian law was in fact compatible with professional monopolization, *if* the framers had accepted the traditional
medieval belief in the power of guilds to minimize prices
through self-imposed regulatory power.

This period is one of transition between a faith in guilds
and the modern belief that monopolization leads to inflated
prices, and the positions of these legislators is somewhat
uncertain. Within a context of faith in guilds, this legislation
is a compensation for the absence of guild regulation: a call
for physicians to charge lower prices or risk state punishment.
In view of the absence of interest-group formation and the
general constraints on local professional monopolization imposed by English incorporation and licensing laws, this compensatory interpretation of the Virginian law seems plausible. It also may have been relatively effective: this act was
apparently satisfactory for a century until a more rationalized (i.e., codified) act setting maximum fees for services was
passed in 1736 by the Virginian Assembly. This bill specifically attacked the "excessive fees" and "unreasonable prices
for the medicines" which physicians charged, and then set
up separate fee tables for practitioners with and without
degrees in "physic."[15] Yet even if this law were based on
a theory of the desirability of guild-type regulation, it had
a strong potential inhibitory effect on interest-group formation. By setting maximum fees, the Virginia legislature greatly reduced the possibility of fee fixing by medical societies
and thereby removed the economic incentive for practitioners to organize. This inhibitory effect persisted long after

[14] Charles M. Andrews, *The Colonial Period of American History* (New Haven
and London: Yale University Press, 1934), vol. 1, pp. 210-211.

[15] Wyndham B. Blanton, *Medicine in Virginia in the Eighteenth Century* (Richmond: Carrett & Massie, 1931), pp. 399-400.

the colonial period ended; unlike the great majority of states, Virginia provided for no medical licensing until 1887.[16]

The irony of this antimonopolistic law, perhaps based on a felt need for compensatory regulation in the absence of monopolization, is that the Virginia Burgesses were intruding on the regulatory monopoly claimed by the Royal College of Physicians. Contained in this law, then, are some of the seeds of political autonomy which were to become increasingly important in colonial affairs. In this case, colonial administration constituted an unavoidable decentralization of authority which favored the development of local regulatory laws that conflicted with English jurisdiction at a number of points.

Other seventeenth-century American laws also appear compatible with a faith in the desirability of guild regulation, but under the circumstances also had a discouraging effect on interest-group formation. A Massachusetts law of 1649 at first appears to have supported the principle of guild regulation when it prohibited anyone from practice who did not follow "the known approved rules of art, in each mistery or occupation" or who acted "(no, not in the most difficult and desperate cases) without the advice and consent of such as are skillful in the same art (if such may be had) or at least of some of the wisest and gravest then present." A New York law of 1664 enacted this Massachusetts law almost word for word.[17] This law, which appears to favor guild formation, in fact discouraged it locally within the context of preexisting English guild privileges. Since licentiates of the RCP were in short supply in seventeenth-century colonial America, a vacuum was created which was favorable to the domination interests of the ruling clergy. And despite the mention of a "mistery" (i.e., guild) in the 1649 law in Massachusetts, there indeed appears to be some evidence that many of the Puritan rulers of the colony, none of them guild members, were themselves active medical practitioners. Oliver Wendell Holmes' review of the history of the medical

[16] Reginald H. Fitz, "The Legislative Control of Medical Practice," *Boston Medical and Surgical Journal* 130 (June 1894), p. 613.
[17] Shafer, *op. cit.*, p. 205.

profession in Massachusetts mentions the scarcity of regularly educated physicians in Massachusetts during the mid-seventeenth century but adds "there were many clergymen who took charge of the bodies as well as the souls of their patients." These clergymen included a large number of the local rulers of the colonies: two presidents of Harvard College (Charles Chauncy and Leonard Hoar), Roger Williams and Anne Hutchinson (both later to leave the Bay Colony to found Rhode Island), three or four generations of Winthrops (including possibly Governor John Winthrop of Massachusetts, definitely his son Governor John Winthrop of Connecticut, Waitstill Winthrop, and Waitstill's son John), and Cotton Mather. In fact, Cotton Mather is remembered by medical historians for his substantial contribution to the curtailment of smallpox in America and Europe by virtue of his revival of interest in variolation, the precursor of vaccination, which employed the smallpox virus variola instead of vaccinia. These men knew of the medical works of major English physicians such as Sydenham, yet, as Holmes points out, they frequently ignored much of the knowledge which was available to them.[18] He attributes this to their interpretation of illness as a manifestation of sinfulness; they were thus caught in the clergyman's habit of "dealing with things unseen; which knowledge and way of thought are special means granted by providence, and to be thankfully accepted."[19] The political implication of Holmes' observations is the conflict between monopolizing impulses on the part of "regular" physicians and of a theocratic regime, both of whom claimed to possess special knowledge and qualification in the same area. The law of 1649 apparently does not benefit either over the other in theory but does set both off from those who in contemporary terms were without "education." In practice, however, the 1649 law favored the theocratic rulers by giving them the legal right to provide for the worldly benefits of their congregations with their own hands. There is a selective monopolism

[18] Oliver Wendell Holmes, *Medical Essays, 1842-1882* (Boston & New York: Houghton, Mifflin, 1889), p. 359.

[19] *Ibid.*, p. 364.

in the 1649 law, which seems to imply that medical practice
should be performed by those with education, but which does
not yet go so far as to permit local specialists in medical
knowledge to control practice. Implicit in this type of
monopolism is the belief that a separate medical monopoly
is unnecessary, for divine knowledge is sufficient or at least
best, and that in any case a separate monopoly would
undermine the legitimacy of the theocracy. Despite the
reference to "mistery" with its nod of recognition of the
RCP's authority, there are substantial glimmerings of autonomy from English rule in the so-called "angelic conjunction"
of medicine and clergy. In the absence of regular guild
members, the failure to secularize medicine in the colonies
inhibited the formation of an interest group of practitioners,
but also went a step further in dissociating the colonies from
English control under the aegis of religious freedom and
responsibility.

Another practice of seventeenth-century colonial legislatures which tended to discourage interest-group formation
was the practice of licensing individual practitioners. Connecticut (1652), Rhode Island (1654), and New York (1677)
and reportedly others issued these licenses. They amounted
to no more than commendations by the colonial legislators,
were given only to long established practitioners of repute,
and carried no penalties for unlicensed practice. They were
intended to encourage good practitioners rather than discourage bad ones, and their value was fundamentally honorific.[20] They discouraged interest-group formation by providing
status rewards without the need for professional organization
and by permitting nonprofessionals to extend official recognition of the quality of certain professionals, that is, to permit
laymen to judge professionals. Yet there was some question
as to the legality of issuing such licenses in view of the legal
constraints discussed, and so the very fact that they were
issued stands out as another example of growing autonomy
from English rule.

While licensing by colonial legislatures may have consti-

[20] Joseph F. Kett, *The Formation of the American Medical Profession: The Role
of Institutions, 1780-1860* (New Haven and London: Yale University Press, 1968),
p. 7.

tuted part of the political break from England prior to the Revolution, it did not contribute to guild formation. The first licensing law, passed in 1760 in New York City, prohibited practice unless previously "examined by one of the Council, the Judge of the Supreme Court, the King's Attorney General and the Mayor or any three of them," and permitted these examiners to proceed as they saw fit. Penalties for violation consisted of a fine of fifty pounds per offense.[21] In New Jersey the legislature established the first provincial system for licensing in 1772 but did not place responsibility in the hands of the medical society. The New Jersey Medical Society, only recently founded in 1766, submitted a petition to the legislature in behalf of regulatory legislation which requested:

That the Profession of a Physician or Surgeon may be reduced to such a Standard of Certainty with Regard to his knowledge, capacity and ability in the several branches, as can instill him or them to practice the same occasionally, UPON THE WHOLE that such mode of Examination may be prescribed, such Forfeitures and Penalties Annexed, and such Testimonials required, and the practice in general so regulated, as in your wisdom you shall think proper to direct.[22]

The legislature saw fit to place regulation in the hands of the government. The judges of the Supreme Court were required to examine and license for practice would-be physicians and surgeons with the advice of "such proper Person or Persons as they in their Discretion shall think fit."[23] This act was reenacted in 1783 with the trivial change that advice should be taken from "two able and skillful practitioners in Physic and Surgery."[24]

---

[21] Shafer, *op. cit.*, pp. 205-206.

[22] Mildred V. Naylor, "A New Jersey Petition," *Bulletin of the History of Medicine* 17 (1945), p. 100.

[23] David L. Cowen, *Medicine and Health in New Jersey: A History* (Princeton, N.J.: D. Van Nostrand Company, 1964), p. 14.

[24] Walter Lincoln Burrage, *A History of the Massachusetts Medical Society, 1781-1922* (Privately printed, 1923), p. 10.

While placing licensure in the hands of the New Jersey government may have been based on contemporary legal concepts, apparently objection specifically to certain monopolistic features of the medical society played a role. This medical society was the first to organize on a colony-wide basis in America, though medical societies had been founded in a number of cities. Its first official action following the creation of an internal government was the creation of "A Table of Fees and Rates" designed to prevent disputes between physicians and patients and to prevent price cutting. It permitted a member to "abate what part of such bills he may think proper, on account of poverty, friendship, or other laudable motives," but "he was 'under pain of expulsion' if such abatement arose from any other consideration whatever."[25] Even though no mention of licensing rights was made for a short time, the very proposal of a minimum fee schedule aroused public opposition. The minutes of the second meeting of the New Jersey Medical Society mentioned that:

"Some evil-minded persons had thrown an odium on the proceedings of this Society, tending to prejudice the minds of the inhabitants against so laudable an Institution. And it was reported to the Board, that the principle clamour of the inhabitants was owing to some improper expression having escaped some member of this Society, in regard to visiting fees and other charges which had brought the Society into disrepute with many persons who esteem it an unjust scheme invented by the Society to bring the inhabitants to terms."[26]

At first the medical society attempted to publish its constitution in public "that thereby a general clamour may be prevented, and that judicious and well-disposed people may have an opportunity to assert and vindicate the propriety of the scheme, and the Legislature be induced to favor it."[27]

[25] Cowen, *op. cit.* (n. 23, above), pp. 11-12.
[26] Burrage, *op. cit.*, pp. 8-9.
[27] Naylor, "New Jersey Petition," p. 93.

The medical society, however, soon withdrew its Table of Fees and Rates and did not reinstate it again until 1786.[28]

The connection between fee tables and licensing laws is particularly important because of the economic futility of attempting fee fixing without adequate restriction of membership and control of members' conduct. While judicial licensing somewhat restricted membership, it did not permit direct, or even indirect, practitioner domination for probably many years. The type of organizational arrangement desired by the New Jersey Medical Society and the absence of organizational recommendations in the society's petition are not clearly explained. The possibility that licensing powers were not placed in medical-society hands along the lines of guild privilege because of antimonopolistic sentiments must be seriously entertained, even though there is no firm evidence that such was the case.

The New Jersey case represents a number of "firsts" which should be cited. It was the first colony-wide medical society in America, and the first medical society to create a fee table and thus encompass economic conduct within its official aims. City medical societies had formed in Boston in 1735 and in New York City in 1749, but only for sharing medical information. Status interests had been included in a 1765 attempt to form a medical society in Massachusetts to improve the prestige of regular physicians over "empirics," i.e., domestic practicioners. Its tactics included not condemning fellow members in public—indeed, preferably not at all— and not stealing patients during consultations. But only a few meetings were held, interest lagged, and the society came to naught.[29] The New Jersey Medical Society was also the first medical society on record to request licensing laws from a local legislature. It was also the first to be criticized on the basis of the economic consequences of what would now be called monopolization, indeed, specifically out of fear of being brought to terms by the organized profession.

That the provincial medical society might have seen the New Jersey arrangement as less than ideal is suggested by

[28] Burrage, op. cit., p. 10.
[29] Ibid., pp. 1-7.

Burrage's report of two "lessons" learned by the Massachusetts Medical Society from the New Jersey incident, as he
relates in his 1923 history of the Massachusetts Medical
Society: "... first, that a state medical society should have
nothing to do with fee tables, they being local affairs to be
sponsored, if at all, by the smaller medical societies in the
different cities and towns of a state; second, for the state
medical society to furnish or control the laws governing the
practice of medicine."[30] He then cites the problem of permitting judges to license physicians: in his own time, some judges
had "considered practitioners of Christian Science or Chiro-
practors as able and skillful. How could they form an intelligent opinion without a knowledge of the principles of the
science of medicine?"[31] The problem appears to have been
obtaining practitioner-controlled licensing by medical societies in the face of public fear of the monopolistic consequences of such arrangements. The choice thus created was
between foregoing economic control devices like fee bills for
the sake of practitioner-dominated licensure or of risking loss
of practitioner domination by placing licensure in the hands
of the government for the sake of quieting public hostility
toward monopolies.

Colonial medical organizations never acquired licensing
powers until after the American Revolution, but the idea
that they might was strongly entertained. John Morgan's
1765 attempt to found an intercolonial licensing medical
society, modeled after the Royal College of Physicians in
London, to be located in Philadelphia ran into opposition
on various levels, and finally failed. Morgan had returned
from schooling at the medical college in Edinburgh with the
highest honors of the day, and in keeping with what appears
to have been a generous dose of egotism, decided to create
a world of status honors similar to those in which he had
received his education. His biographer has detailed how
Morgan's desire for prestige and personal control of all
organized medical activities in America contributed to both

[30] *Ibid.*, p. 12.
[31] *Ibid.*

Morgan's successes and difficulties.[32] He succeeded in founding the first American medical school in Philadelphia and established the so-called "regular mode of practice" as the dominant type of orthodox medical education in the New World. This regular mode was a derivation from a systematization of medical theory by William Cullen at Edinburgh (the same Cullen who clashed with Adam Smith), which had been brought to the colonies by Morgan and a number of other American students who went to Edinburgh and which had been continued after the American Revolution by Morgan's student Benjamin Rush. It was this association of the institutions of medical orthodoxy with the regular mode of practice which led to the adoption of the appellation of "regular" for Establishment medical organizations.

But while Morgan was successful in promulgating a prestigious institution of education in Pennsylvania, he failed in organizing the profession. Shryock cites the conventional opinion that the failure was due to the preexisting monopoly held by the Royal College in London and to the advice given to the Penns, the proprietors, that such an institution should not be chartered.[33] This interpretation ignores the fact that the licensing plan was seriously considered for some time by the Penns. Presumably the rapidly growing sense of local American autonomy provided for some leeway. Morgan's biographer suggests some of the complexity of the situation. Some of the ruling figures of Pennsylvania were reportedly favorable to the idea. The Chief Justice and John Penn were impressed by the potential for honor for the province, but others persuaded Thomas Penn against the plan. The provost of the College of Philadelphia warned against weakening the medical department at the College by activating feuds between Morgan and other contenders for medical power in the city. The famous physician John Fothergill, a personal friend of Morgan's in London, agreed in a letter to Penn that there was indeed lack of unanimity over the plan in

---

[32] Whitfield J. Bell, Jr., *John Morgan: Continental Doctor* (Philadelphia: University of Pennsylvania Press, 1965).

[33] Richard Harrison Shryock, *Medical Licensing in America, 1650-1965* (Baltimore: Johns Hopkins Press, 1967), p. 17.

Philadelphia, and added an attack against medical monopolies in general:

> There is a College of Physicians at Edinburgh, at Paris, in London, and other places. Experience does not clearly prove they have been of much utility. The pretence of founding these Societies was to countenance and support the regular Physician, to suppress Quackery; but the effect has generally ended in a sort of monopoly. A few have got into the management of these Societies, who have gradually found means in order to raise themselves, and lay others, not less knowing, able or honest, under great difficulties. All the advantages of a medical Society may be obtained without a Charter. There has been one in London several years, unconnected with the College, that has communicated more useful knowledge to the world, than the colleges have done in their corporate capacity, since the time of their first foundation.[34]

Fothergill's bitter comments are a reminder of the sources of antimonopolistic thought in the rationalist Enlightenment, which distrusted the tendencies of monopolies to promote restricted access to secret knowledge rather than to augment the body of knowledge. This distrust had also been expressed by Gregory with respect to ethics. Fothergill may well have also had personal reason to distrust the college system, since as a Quaker he had allegedly been denied access to a degree from Cambridge or Oxford and had therefore been admitted to the RCP of London only as a Licentiate and not as a prestigious fellow.[35] Nonetheless, Fothergill's argument is instructive of the way in which rationalist thought could lead away from the conventional monopolistic assumptions within the organized profession. A few months after Penn's refusal to charter Morgan's proposal, the Philadelphia Medical Society "merged in the American Society for Promoting Useful Knowledge and lost its identity."[36] The

[34] Bell, *op. cit.*, pp. 138-140.
[35] George W. Corner, *Two Centuries of Medicine* (Philadelphia and Montreal: J. B. Lippincott, 1965), p. 30.
[36] Bell, *op. cit.*, p. 140.

experience may well have been historically traumatic; as in the case of Virginia, no licensing law was passed in Pennsylvania until 1893.[37]

As Americans gradually developed a sense of autonomy from England, eventually culminating in the Revolution, preexisting English legal constraints began to weaken their hold. The common law restriction on chartering of corporations by corporations appears to have been maintained, although in certain cases such as the proprietory colony of Pennsylvania, incorporation of a medical society with licensing powers was briefly considered. The monopoly on licensing held by the Royal College of Physicians was not uncommonly ignored by colonial legislatures, but the power of licensing was retained in the hands of government officials, i.e., in the courts, the executive, and the legislature. There was some development of medical interest groups, but they were able to gain little apparent control of the situation, and their history is mostly one of practitioner disinterest, due to powerlessness, and shortlived existence. There is some evidence for the existence of antimonopolistic sentiments toward medical organizations, but their role is difficult to ascertain, since any effect they might have had was in the same direction as legal constraints. In those cases in which legal constraints weakened, however, antimonopolistic beliefs may well have played some part in restraining the development of medical monopolization.

The period of special incorporation laws (1776-1837)

After the American Revolution the situation rapidly reversed due to the new legal status of the former colonial provinces and their liberation from English statutory law. The colonies which had formerly been English corporations became states and were then free to charter corporations under common law (which had not been suspended in the new nation). The RCP's legal monopoly on licensing was no longer binding following liberation from the domination of the English parliament, for the medical monopoly had been based on statutory law. Throughout the new states,

[37] Fitz, "Legislative Control," p. 613.

medical societies were rapidly chartered, incorporated, and given a variety of powers. Certain medical societies approximated the ideal monopolization strategy to a remarkable degree, particularly those which adopted the organizational structure of the old English RCP. Yet the degree of monopolization attained by these early state medical societies was, overall, highly variable.

With the decline of legal restraints on medical monopolization, antimonopolistic forces became more important determinants of professional structures. Antimonopolistic feeling was not directed primarily at medical practitioners; but when the situation was appropriate, general antimonopolistic arguments were made against the medical societies as well. Therefore, to understand the relationship between the rise of antimonopolistic ideologies and the rise of professional organizations, one should examine what was happening in larger American society. Despite objections to monopoly, the medical profession occasionally succeeded in establishing a few practitioner-dominated organizations. Yet in the process, medical organizations gained a popular reputation as monopolistic, and as will be seen, this term was politically employed in a hostile fashion.

The incorporation of medical societies soon after the Revolution (Table 1) was opposed by antimonopolistic ideologies

Table 1

Incorporation of State Medical Societies

Date	Incorporated Societies
1781	Massachusetts
1788	New York
1789	Delaware, South Carolina
1791	New Hampshire
1792	Connecticut
1799	Maryland
1800	North Carolina
1804	Georgia
1913	Rhode Island, Vermont
1824	Virginia

Source: W. B. McDaniel, II, "A Brief Sketch of the Rise of American Medical Societies," in History of American Medicine: A Symposium (Edited by Felix Marti-Ibanez, New York: MD Publications, 1958), pp. 138–139.

directed at the political uses of corporations in general.
For example, a petition for incorporation of a state medical
society delivered to the Connecticut legislature by delegates
of the Medical Society of New Haven County in 1785 was
refused because of suspicion of the motives of the petitioners,
"some ignorant and ill-minded persons having misrepre-
sented their designs, and insinuated that the main object
was to increase the pecuniary emoluments of the faculty."[38]
The petition was rewritten, and arguments were prepared
about the use of incorporated medical societies by other state
governments and "enlightened nations." A bill introduced
in 1787 for this purpose did not, however, pass the upper
house of the legislature. Antimonopolistic feelings played a
manifest part in this rejection:

> In explanation of the hostile action of the assembly,
> it may be said that it was not then customary to make
> laws for the benefit, or seeming benefit, of particular
> classes. There was a well-grounded apprehension of
> danger which might come from special privileges and
> monopoly. In 1787 a few cities had been recently incor-
> porated, but what may be called a private charter did
> not (I believe) exist in the state. Very naturally, the
> legislature was reluctant to change its policy. More than
> this, there were provisions in the rejected bill calculated
> to excite the jealousy of a suspicious people. I refer
> particularly to those parts of the act which gave to the
> corporators and members the right to choose their asso-
> ciates and successors, and to the society the power to
> disfranchise (professionally) and impose pecuniary pen-
> alties, &c.[39]

Public discussion of the issue occurred; the seniors of Yale
College debated the question "Whether it be safe to grant
the proposed charter of the Connecticut Medical Society?"
and some months later the question "Whether the institution

[38] Henry Bronson, "Historical Account of the Origin of the Connecticut Medical
Society," *Proceedings of Connecticut Medical Society* (May 1873), pp. 55-56.
[39] *Ibid.*, pp. 58-59.

of medical societies be useful?" Unfortunately, no record of their arguments or conclusions remains, though one observer claims that keen public interest "developed from the fear lest chartering a medical society might create a private monopoly."[40]

In 1792, a bill of incorporation finally passed into law after the Medical Society of New Haven County had rephrased its purpose as the creation of a medical library. Powers of examination, licensing, fines, and dues were denied to the newly incorporated state society.[41] In 1800, the state medical society quietly assumed licensing powers, but apparently antimonopolism had already played a major role in drastically curtailing medical monopolization. There were, for example, no penalties for violations.

The word "monopoly" carried a different meaning then than we understand today, and to appreciate this difference, one should examine the political context in which it appeared. Special incorporation laws did not prohibit or restrict trade or activities in any particular sphere; rather, they only permitted particular (special) parties to enjoy the benefits of incorporation. Without being restrictive, they afforded the recipients of charters a more favorable position of domination in the market and, in some cases, made possible activities impossible without incorporation privileges, such as limited liability, joint stock ownership, and so forth. Under special incorporation laws, then, the government made substantial gifts of ecomonic power to particular individuals and groups without infringing on traditional freedoms of trade. Anyone could legally compete with corporations if he so pleased. Nonetheless, these laws gave rise to the fear that the government would further concentrate national wealth into the hands of the already wealthy. Alexander Hamilton's federalist mercantilism was a philosophy of the time which explicitly asserted that government's responsibility was to help the activities of the wealthy, stating that the wealthy had the most to lose and the most with which to accomplish objec-

[40] Walter Ralph Steiner, *The Evolution of Medicine in Connecticut, with the Foundation of the Yale Medical School as its Notable Achievement* (No publisher, 1914), pp. 7-8.
[41] Bronson, "Historical Account," p. 62.

tives. Corporate laws were seen as one instrument of Hamiltonian federalism and so became the target of certain groups whose interests were threatened.[42]

During the first quarter-century after the Revolution, the strategy for meeting this threat underwent a change in response to changing conditions. In the beginning, prior to the establishment of corporations, some hoped to prevent their creation. This hope resulted in an antimonopolistic ideology directed at *all* corporations and raised the prospect of a society without corporate bodies. When this strategy failed and corporations, particularly business corporations, were successfully established, a new strategy of democratizing incorporation privileges arose. Instead of attempting to eliminate corporations, ascendent interest groups attacking the favorable power position of established wealth apparently settled for trying to extend corporate privileges to themselves as well. They came to see corporate privileges as a new potential means for upward mobility rather than as an obstacle. Revised antimonopolistic ideologies focusing on the special nature of incorporation laws gave birth to the idea of general incorporation laws as part of this attack. Incorporation advantages would be deemed permissible, but no particular group was supposed to monopolize them. The first of these two strategies is generally known to historians as the anticorporation movement, the second as Jacksonian democracy. Yet they were two reactions to the same challenge: the spector of federalist mercantilism.

The anticorporation branch of antifederalism had adopted the accusation of monopoly as one of its ideological tools, directing the charge at all corporations. The main argument against permitting the concentration of wealth as a consequence of corporate privileges was that it would subvert political democracy:

> One legislator voiced this fear: "If the legislature may mortgage, or, in other words, charter away portions of either the privileges or powers of the state—if they may

[42] Arthur M. Schlesinger, *The Age of Jackson* (Boston: Little, Brown, 1945), pp. 179-182.

incorporate bodies for the sole purpose of gain, with the power of making by-laws, and of enjoying the emolument of privilege, profit, influence, or power—and cannot disannul their own deed, and restore to the citizens their right of equal protection, power, privilege and influence—the consequence is, that some foolish and wanton assembly may parcel out the commonwealth into little aristocracies, and so overturn the nature of our government without remedy."[43]

The anticorporation spokesmen feared that the government would not reserve the right to withdraw incorporation charters, thereby making legally privileged groups irrevocably permanent. They thus feared a wide variety of types of corporations: societies of tradesmen and mechanics, the Connecticut Medical Society in 1787, the Bank of North America in 1785-87, and others.[44] Despite vocal opposition, corporations flourished and criticism declined after 1792 as more experience with corporations was acquired. Slowly a distinction was beginning to be drawn between business and nonbusiness corporations: "It is probably fair to say that the broader opposition rested on traditional antipathy to such corporations as the closed corporations of the English boroughs, the restrictive guilds, and the monopolistic companies for foreign trade; and that the American business corporation turned out to be quite a different sort of creature."[45] Granted, much of this change in attitude was due to the discovery that certain useful enterprises such as bridge and canal building could only be done by corporations able to concentrate sufficient capital for the job. But the success of incorporation law should also be ascribed to the political power of the established wealthy and their interest in securing corporate advantages for themselves. In any event, anticorporation forces could not mobilize adequate political opposition, and corporations became established features of American organizational life.

[43] J. Davis, op. cit. (n. 12, above), vol. II, p. 304.
[44] Ibid., pp. 303-307.
[45] Ibid., p. 309.

The anticorporation movement affected the organization of the medical profession in a variety of ways. Table 2 presents a cumulative picture of the state of medical licensing in the United States prior to 1850. Unfortunately, not all of the information is available to complete the picture, but some insights can be obtained from it even as is. Legal authority for licensure was placed in various hands: county and state *medical societies* adopted the guild principle by holding examinations and issuing licenses in New York, New Jersey, Rhode Island, New Hampshire, Massachusetts, Delaware, the District of Columbia, Ohio, Indiana, and Michigan. *State boards* were established first in Maryland, then in South Carolina, Georgia, Alabama, Mississippi, Louisiana, and Tennessee. In most of these, state board members were appointed by either the state legislature or the governor, but in at least one state—Maryland—they were appointed by the state medical society. In two cases, Connecticut and Maine, licensing powers were held by a *conjoint board consisting of the state medical society and a medical college.* As one can see, the more southern states were least likely to provide guildlike authority to the state medical societies. Indeed, during the first quarter of the nineteenth century, Pennsylvania, Virginia, and North Carolina provided for no medical licensing, and the last two of these were firmly within the southern sphere. Probably these differences can best be accounted for by the relative strength of Hamiltonian federalism in the northeastern states, where legislatures were most receptive to the idea of placing licensing powers in the hands of those private parties whose interests were most immediately affected. Yet there were exceptions. In the South, some substantial professional control of licensing was acquired in Maryland by letting medical societies appoint the membership of state licensing boards. In the North, New Jersey created a system of district boards in place of medical society licensing in 1830.

Restrictions on unlicensed practitioners varied in scope. Unlicensed practice per se was prohibited in most states, but in some states such as Connecticut and Massachusetts, unlicensed practitioners were prohibited only from suing for

Table 2

Early Medical Licensing Legislation in the United States

State	Year of Passage	Licensing Agency	Restrictions on the Unlicensed	Fines; Other Penalties	Exemptions	Year of Repeal
New York	1806	state/county societies	fee collection prohibited	1807: $5; 1812: $25 (suspended 1813–1827) 1827: imprisonment	1806: diploma 1807:herbalists 1827: Regent's diploma	1844
New Jersey	1816	1816: county societies 1818: state societies; examination by county societies 1830: three district boards	fee collection, unlicensed practice prohibited	$25	1851: graduates of certain medical schools in New York and Pennsylvania 1854: diploma	1864
Connecticut	1800	conjoint board of medical college and medical society	1800: suing for fees prohibited	—	—	1842
Maine	1821	conjoint board of medical college and society	1830: unlicensed practice prohibited	—	—	—
Rhode Island	1812	state or district board	—	—	—	—

New Hampshire		state or district board	—	—	—	—
Massachusetts	1781	state or district society	1818: suing for fees prohibited	—	1818: diploma from incorporated medical college	1835
Maryland	1799	state board composed of 12 members, elected by state medical society	1801: unlicensed practice, suing for fees prohibited	1801: $50 per offense	diploma waives examination requirement	1838
Georgia	1826 1839	"board of physicians"	unlicensed practice prohibited	$500	1839: "Thomsonian or Botanic practice, or any other practitioner of medicine in this state."	1835
Alabama	1823	five state boards —each with three members elected by state legislature	unlicensed practice prohibited	$500	diploma	? 1831, ? 1833
Mississippi	—	three state boards appointed by state legislature	unlicensed practice prohibited	$500; imprisonment to six months	—	1834

Source: Kett, *op. cit.*, pp. 181–184; N. S. Davis, *Medical Education*, pp. 88–105; Steiner, *op. cit.*, p. 8.

Table 2 (Continued)

State	Year of Passage	Licensing Agency	Restrictions on the Unlicensed	Fines; Other Penalties	Exemptions	Year of Repeal
Louisiana	1820	two boards, six members each, appointed by governor	unlicensed practice prohibited	first offense: $100 second offense: $200, imprisonment to one year	diploma	—
Tennessee	1830	a board	—	none	—	—
District of Columbia	1819	state board	unlicensed practice, suing for fees prohibited	$50 per offense	diploma	—
Delaware	1822	state board	unlicensed practice, suing for fees prohibited	$50 per offense	diploma	—
Ohio	1812	state, county, and district medical societies	unlicensed practice, suing for fees prohibited	yes	1818: diploma	1833 (also repeal of incorporation law)

Indiana, Michigan	1840's	diploma	yes	unlicensed practice, suing for fees prohibited	state, county, district medical	—
South Carolina	1838	diploma	$500; imprisonment to two months	unlicensed practice, suing for fees prohibited	two districts	1817

fees. For a time New York and New Jersey both prohibited collecting fees for unlicensed practice, but did not prohibit practice per se. New York in time extended restrictions to practice in general. Maryland, the District of Columbia, Delaware, South Carolina, Ohio, Indiana, and Michigan all made a point of prohibiting both unlicensed practice and suing for fees.

Penalties for violations were more severe in the more southern states. Fines in New York and New Jersey varied from 5 to 25 dollars, but in Maryland, the District of Columbia, and Delaware, ran 50 dollars per offense. Except for Louisiana, which carried 100 and 200 dollar fines, most of the remaining southern states with licensing laws carried stiff fines of 500 dollars. The major exception, Tennessee, applied no penalties. In general, imprisonment was applied only in southern states, though New York also adopted it in 1827.

In retrospect, the weakest licensing laws were probably those which most closely emulated the English guilds and allowed the most monopolization of medical practice. In Massachusetts, for instance, medical societies issued licenses, but for thirty-seven years following the institution of licensing, no restrictions of any sort were placed on unlicensed practitioners. When introduced, restrictions amounted to no more than not suing for fees, an easily evaded prohibition which was occasionally challenged successfully in the courts. Apparently the prohibition had been instituted by the Massachusetts legislature without request by the medical society; in 1835 it was removed because the Massachusetts Medical Society believed it afforded popular sympathy to unlicensed practitioners, who were made to appear persecuted.[46] New York provided restrictions but did not penalize unlicensed practice between 1813 and 1827.[47] New York's laws were further complicated by the exemption of a wide class of practitioners from the licensing requirement. Practice was open to any "persons using, for the benefit of the sick, any

[46] Kett, op. cit. (n. 20, above), p. 16.
[47] James J. Walsh, History of Medicine in New York: Three Centuries of Medical Progress (New York: National Americana Society, 1919), vol. I, pp. 83-85.

roots or herbs, the growth of the United States," beginning
the year following the establishment of licensing provisions.
This exemption was discarded between 1827 and 1830, and
removed again in part between 1834 and 1835; but it was
in general a provision which made the rest of the law virtually
worthless as a means for restricting membership. It legalized
practice by the numerous domestic herbalist practitioners,
which constituted the major source of competition to the
regular profession for many years.

Exemptions from these laws were so common that the
system of licensure became only one among many portals
of entry into the profession. The New York case of exemptions for domestic practitioners—echoed in Georgia in 1839—
should not obscure the more common and important alternative to entry: medical school diplomas. The incorporation
of medical societies had preceded the incorporation of medical schools by several years, but as teaching institutions
appeared, legislatures accepted them as well as licensing
bodies. The existence of this multiple portal system was later
to spell a crucial threat to the continuance of the medical
societies, a problem that will be taken up later in this chapter.

Monopolization by medical societies during this period,
then, was constrained from several directions. Some states
refused to unite licensing and medical societies; others, which
did, failed to place significant restrictions on unlicensed
practice and did not institute major penalties. All states
reduced restriction of membership in the profession by adding
alternative portals of entry. Finally, one state after another
repealed penalties on unlicensed practice, beginning in the
1830's. Apparently special incorporation laws had been
granted to medical societies during this period only at the
price of curtailing substantial monopolization. In those instances in which medical societies approximated the model
of the English medical guilds, as in the northern states,
antimonopolistic sentiments were so powerful that the power
of licensing could not be used appreciably to the advantage
of the medical societies; a license amounted to little more
than an honorific title. In the southern states, the restrictive
nature of medical licensing appears to have been more

substantial, but there is no evidence that the medical societies exercised appreciable control of the system. So while
restriction of membership in the profession may have occurred, it was apparently not under the domination of
organized practitioners. In the southern states, as well, there
is some evidence of popular suspicion of the monopolistic
tendencies of the medical profession often extending into the
legislatures.[48]

The repeal of licensing penalties and, in the case of Ohio,
of the incorporation of medical societies represents a different
phase in the history of this period. While licensing laws had
permitted incorporation and some measure of restriction of
practice to certain practitioners, repeal left incorporation
alone but reversed restrictionist tendencies. To an extent,
repeals were due to antimonopolistic ideologies, but more
immediately to the declining use of licensing as a means for
ascertaining competence. The argument with respect to the
role of antimonopolistic ideologies requires examination, for
at least one major analyst of this period believes that the
repeal of licensing laws was due to an upsurge of irrational
Jacksonian democracy and populist anti-intellectualism.[49]
That such was not the case is an interesting point in sociological explanation, but also an important part of understanding the development of the American medical profession.

To be sure, Jacksonian democrats attacked corporations
as "monopolies," but one should understand the meaning
of this charge. Unlike the earlier anticorporation movement,
Jacksonian democracy did not launch a wholesale attack
on all corporations. Fear of federalism continued in the form
of opposition to corporations such as the second United
States Bank which threatened to become "oligarchical," i.e.,
too big and powerful. "Monopoly" did not refer to restric-
tiveness; other banks were permitted to exist. "Monopoly"
referred in this context to the legal privileging of one group
with corporate benefits from the government. It "meant no
more than privileges given to *some* which were not freely
open to *all*, rather than privileges assured to some to the

---

[48] Kett, *op. cit.* (n. 20, above), p. 19.
[49] Shryock, *op. cit.* (n. 33, above), p. 31.

exclusion of all others.'[50] To this extent, the use of the concept of monopoly to diagnose the situation had not changed since the postrevolutionary reaction to federalism. But the strategy to deal with monopolies had changed. Instead of focusing on the type of organization which provided a power advantage, and instead of attacking corporations as monopolies, it attacked the monopolization of corporate privileges by certain groups. Instead of trying to abolish a monopoly on corporate privileges, it attempted to expand membership in the monopoly, at least in terms of the number of corporations within any specific sphere of activity. This revised strategy culminated in the development of general rather than special incorporation laws.

In a crucial New Jersey court case, a charter awarded to only one company for construction of a bridge served as the focus for opposition to "monopoly." Supreme Court review of the case in 1837 under the leadership of the Jacksonian Taney supported the view that other companies should also be able to receive such charters, and with this decision general incorporation laws were born.[51] The issuance of a charter to one business organization was not seen as inconsistent with the issuance of a second or more which would result in competition within the same market. In this sense, Jacksonian antimonopolism professed the desirability of corporate competition and thus differed from earlier antimonopolistic beliefs. Indeed, this legal change stimulated corporation building in American business life. Whereas initial reaction to the wealth-enhancing properties of corporations had proposed prohibiting them as unfair and dangerous, later reaction proposed expanding them. From the point of view of the economic interests of *ascendent* wealthy groups, opening up this means of concentrating wealth and power promised to be an important means of upward mobility in their competition with the established wealthy, certainly a more promising strategy than attempting to eliminate corporation.[52]

[50] J. Davis, *op. cit.* (n. 12, above), p. 320.
[51] Schlesinger, *op. cit.*, pp. 324-325, 336-337.
[52] Richard Hofstadter, "Andrew Jackson and the Rise of Liberal Capitalism," in Edwin C. Rozwenc, ed., *The Meaning of Jacksonian Democracy* (Boston: D. C. Heath 1963), pp. 81-92.

The period of general incorporation laws (post 1837)

Any attempt to relate the repeal of medical licensing laws directly to Jacksonian antimonopolistic beliefs shows that these beliefs were not consistent with repeal. Earlier anticorporate sentiment was not relevant, since as has already been mentioned, the corporate status of state medical societies was not repealed except in Ohio. Nor was licensing authority removed from the hands of those medical societies which had received it after the Revolution. The object of attack was the penalties for violation of existing licensing laws. In effect, the restrictive component of medical licensing laws was removed; licenses might still continue to be issued, but no one could be legally restricted from practicing. The differences between this situation and the definition of monopoly used by Jacksonian democrats illustrate why Jacksonian democracy is not an adequate explanation for repeal. First, Jacksonian democracy was directed not at restrictive corporations but at companies privileged by a monopoly on incorporation advantages. True, state medical societies had unique charters, but that does not explain the removal of restrictive penalties. Second, Jacksonian democracy became committed to a strategy of general incorporation laws. The logical consequence would have been the extension of medical licensing to other types of chartered medical societies, as occurred when the Massachusetts Homeopathic Medical Society was incorporated in 1856. Yet this strategy would not have resulted in the removal of penalties.

The relationship of antimonopolistic beliefs to repeal of penalties in medical licensing legislation is very complex indeed. First, there is the problem of timing. Repeal began in 1833 (possibly even in 1831) and swept rapidly through the southern states, which had not vested licensing authority in medical societies. At least two northern states, however, Ohio and Massachusetts, shared in this early period of repeal; therefore, one cannot fully explain it in terms of the absence of dominant federalist groups, which almost certainly played a part in every other case. After 1839, the conversion of federalism into Whiggery helps explain some of the repeals. The political representatives of established wealth in the

nation, the Whig party, had developed a strategy for outdoing
the Democrats electorally with "democratic" gestures, which
a number of historians have regarded as token surrenders
of the principle of privilege for the benefit of popular support.
If not token, at least these political acts would "insure that
reform would come in the shape least distasteful to the
business community."[53] In Maryland, for instance, this strategy worked against the orthodox profession when Whigs
joined with Democrats against grants of exclusive privilege
and gave Thomsonians (a group of irregular practitioners)
the right to sue for fees. While, in general, the medical issue
did not give rise to division along party lines either in
Maryland or any other state,[54] from the point of view of
large business interests, the organized medical profession was
one of those expendable privileged groups which could be
used for electoral gain. If medical licensing rode in under
the cover of ascendent federalism, it rode out with federalism's conversion to Whiggery. In this sense, Jacksonian
democracy did contribute in a small way to the removal of
licensing penalties, but mostly through its stimulation of
Whiggery.

Second, opposition to licensing penalties on the part of
even the medical societies should be contended with. In
Massachusetts, penalties were opposed to prevent activation
of the charge of monopoly among the public.[55] Following
the advent of general incorporation laws, the societies let
the practical importance of licensing decline in the hope that
new competitive medical societies formed by Thomsonians,
eclectics, homeopaths, and other "sectarians" would not be
chartered. Given a choice between restrictive legislation and
a monopoly on chartered incorporation, and in some cases,
on licensing, the regular profession surely did not want to
share its position of official legitimacy. The fear was that,
under general incorporation laws, the argument might be
made that if regulars should be entitled to license practitioners, so should irregulars. In light of professional developments which will be discussed shortly, it was more prudent

[53] Schlesinger, op. cit. (n. 42, above), p. 286.
[54] Kett, op. cit. (n. 20, above), p. 57.
[55] Ibid., p. 16.

to let licensing laws go. Yet the manifest attitude of spokesmen of the profession was that while "voluntarization" was
politically sagacious, they were not very pleased about it.

Third, there was the paradox that the failure of the medical
profession to adequately monopolize during the early nineteenth century only served to validate public animosity
toward existing monopolization. A recent reviewer's attempt
to summarize the considerations entering into repeal provides a platform for demonstrating how this occurred:

> In summary, then, all those factors, the state of medical
> practice, the faculty disputes, the inability of the doctors
> to agree upon diagnosis and treatment, the inferior
> physicians annually "turned loose" upon the communi-
> ty, and the monopolistic tendencies of the profession,
> combined to reduce the prestige and influence of the
> physician. These help to explain the widespread demand
> to repeal the licensure laws, which would break the
> monopoly of orthodox medicine.[56]

While it is clear that patently monopolistic features of the
medical profession, such as restrictive licensing and uniform
fee bills, might have activated antimonopolistic sentiment,
the other factors, though not part of the profession's monopolistic achievements, also activated it. The increase in "inferior physicians" was a direct product of the increase in the
number of medical schools (which had doubled between 1830
and 1850)[57] and of the practice in many states of accepting
medical school diplomas as an alternative to medical society
licenses. Thus, the production of "inferior physicians" was
a result of the organized profession's failure to shut alternative portals of entry into the profession, and of the medical
schools' success in taking advantage of the opportunity.

The existence of internal disputes, such as medical faculty
conflicts and theoretical arguments, along with a low public
opinion of the general state of medical attainment, evidently
gave rise to the question of what public protection was
afforded by providing certain doctors with a monopoly. The

[56] Martin Kaufman, *Homeopathy in America: The Rise and Fall of a Medical
Heresy* (Baltimore and London: Johns Hopkins Press, 1971), p. 50.
[57] *Ibid.*, p. 49.

existence of sectarian competitors who apparently gave no
worse treatment than the orthodox profession also made
restrictive privileges problematic; yet the existence of these
irregulars was itself a failure of the organized profession to
eliminate outside competition. So it can be seen that a
number of the liked and disliked features of medical practice
of the time can in fact be ascribed to the organized profession's *lack* of monopolization. Features which were liked,
such as the relatively popular sectarian competitors, helped
to work against maintaining monopolization. Features which
were disliked, such as inferior physicians, were blamed on
those monopolists, the medical societies.

In retrospect, it would appear that what happened to the
medical societies during this period was highly ironic. The
licensing functions of medical societies, or in certain cases,
their examination functions, declined following the rapid
proliferation of medical schools and practitioners with some
measure of formal medical education. Since most states
accepted medical school diplomas as well as licenses as a
means of satisfying legal requirements for practice, fewer
applications for licenses were made in favor of diplomas. The
medical societies had not successfully restricted entry into
the profession, and their own means of control over entry
was becoming progressively weaker as medical students simply took diplomas. The license was becoming a symbol of
inferior education, since it was taken mainly by those who
were not able to obtain diplomas. Not surprisingly, as the
prestige of licenses declined, so did the number of physicians
who took licenses. This phenomenon is an interesting piece
of evidence against Shryock's belief that anti-intellectual
and antieducational biases of the Jacksonians led to licensing
repeal: medical school diplomas were probably becoming
more acceptable than licenses as evidence of competence in
the medical market. As such, the medical societies were
increasingly seen as privileged institutions inferior to medical
schools. Monopolistic privileges under such circumstances
became increasingly hard to justify, and as the institution
of medical society licensing became a dead horse, the charge
of monopoly became more conspicuous.

The decline of licensing brought three major problems for

the medical societies. The first problem was to find a new political function for the medical societies, one which would further medical society control over practitioners. The second was to subordinate medical schools to the medical societies to protect the interests of organized practitioners. And the third was to escape public accusations of monopoly. The first problem was difficult to solve because of the existence of public charges of monopoly and because of the latent threat that general incorporation laws would prevent the organized practitioners from monopolizing practice by permitting competing medical groups to organize and demand equal rights of control. The second was difficult due to the existence of multiple portals of entry into the profession and easy chartering of medical colleges under the loose general incorporation laws of the period. And the third was difficult to solve, since most traditional means of group control were readily recognized as monopolistic. The need was for a strategy of domination of the profession by the medical societies which would deny both control and monopolization—or at least make them less conspicuous and easily identified—yet permit them to take place.

The facade of demonopolization was pursued by three techniques. The first was the voluntarization of medical society membership. Prior to 1844, membership in a medical society and licensure were linked, frequently by law, most commonly in the northern states. Following the repeal in New York of the legal requirement of compulsory membership in a medical society for all licensed physicians, medical societies did not demand this unification. The decline in the number of physicians taking licenses, of course, simply made such laws irrelevant. The second technique was the argument that the medical profession did not require legal privileges to protect its own interests. As one prominent New York physician wrote:

The medical profession, let the people understand, is not dependent on the protection of law, and it comes not to their hall of legislation to beg any favor. It can have its own organization, and stand upon its own character alone. If the charter should be surrendered, and the plan of voluntary association should be adopted in full, renouncing all dependence upon law, those who entered into it would probably enjoy as much emolument from the practice of medicine as they now do.[58]

This defense of motives was accompanied, however, by a suggestion that it would be in the self-interest of the community to defend itself from "irregular and irresponsible practitioners," who would multiply in the absence of laws.[59]

The third technique was a newly acquired faith in the capacity of the medical profession under a voluntary system to mobilize favorable public opinion through traditional ethical regulations. Hooker, as late as 1844, argued that physicians were unpopular because they erringly tried to curry public favor by adopting the tactics of empirics, i.e., domestic practitioners: "Like the most arrant quack, the unwise physician yields to the caprice and whims of the multitude to gain their favor. When he does this he inflicts a wound upon the honor of the profession; and, by bringing it down from its noble and elevated calling to a competition with empiricism, essentially degrades it in the eyes of the community."[60] Reputable members of the profession were supposed to remedy this by augmenting the honor of the profession and standing above the empirics. Communion with empiricism in any form was to be suspended; competition should be honorable (physicians should not advance their own reputations in public or denounce other physicians), "an honorable *esprit de corps*" should be cultivated, and "temporary emolument must be given up whenever required to advance the interests of the whole."[61] In short, the profession should adhere to the principles of "medical police," i.e., medical ethics. Medical societies would function in building favorable public opinion by allowing physicians to disengage

[58] Worthington Hooker, *Dissertation on the Respect Due to the Medical Profession and the Reasons that It is Not Awarded By the Community* (Norwich, Conn.: J. G. Pooley, 1844), pp. 27-28.
[59] *Ibid.*
[60] *Ibid.*, p. 15.
[61] *Ibid.*, pp. 17, 22.

themselves from claims of superior medical efficacy (at which "quacks" frequently got the better of them) and by permitting them to appeal to their reputation among fellow physicians.

Hooker's program, or interpretation of what was happening, was unrealistic in a number of senses. First, it relied on changing public desiderata from evidence of medical efficacy to professional testimony; why the public would be willing to do this was not explained. Second, it attempted to increase public popularity by dissociation from the techniques of popular practitioners. How this would work was similarly unexplained. In fact, claims of superior honor might well have antagonized the public by appearing to be yet another medical pretension. Third, Hooker was naive to state that the interests of the profession did not require legal protection. Without legal restraints, the number of practitioners could be expected to increase to some extent, and competition would likely increase.

Yet Hooker's program may not have been meant to be realistic. It was concerned with disengaging the profession from charges of monopoly acquired during a half century of licensing privileges. Nothing could be more consistent with popular libertarian conceptions of consumer sovereignty than claiming to pursue power through public relations building. The medical societies in this plan would be no more than scientific bodies and public-relations offices for practitioners. And it permitted some physicians to believe that the path to success was through "ethics" and other demonstrations of integrity. Hooker's plan was pointedly directed at physicians for an audience. It was an attack on the irrationality of the public and served to make physicians self-defensive and mutually protective against the public. As such, it was an ideology designed to build internal solidarity in the face of social changes which seemed difficult to comprehend.

As a diagnosis of the times, Hooker's interpretation was inaccurate. He ascribed the decline of licensing privileges to irrational public preference for "hordes" of quacks, and in this he was mistaken. The largest problem for the organ-

ized profession came from the sudden and dramatic proliferation of regular physicians from new medical schools. To
this extent, Hooker's work was not a rational contribution
to a better monopolization strategy, but it did form part
of that strategy by directing attention away from areas in
which the organized profession began to establish indirect
dominative relationships.

Indirect de facto domination was established over the next
several decades in a number of different settings, as the
organized profession explored new avenues of control following its failure at monopolization through licensure. Control
over hiring practices by medical school faculties, public
hospitals, the army medical corps, and governmental commissions was increased by de facto domination of agency
examining boards and, when necessary, by wholesale resignations and boycotts in protest over the hiring of homeopaths
and other competitors to the orthodox profession.[62] Another
development was the increasing domination over the curriculum provided by medical schools, the means of which were
at this time limited to persuasive appeals. These new control
devices were exceptions to a program of altering public
opinion by using ethical claims, but they did not constitute
examples of monopolization in contemporaneously recognizable terms, that is, as legal privileges. They were monopoli-
zations of the administration of nonprofessional institutions
with respect to the regulation of professional activity. They
did not require favorable public opinion—except in a noninterventionist sense—or particularly attract public opposition,
because they did not fit into the imagery of salient popular
ideologies of domination, even though they permitted indirect domination and, as in these examples, some measure
of monopolization.

Yet even these indirect measures were not very effective
means of monopolization. The most important development
toward more effective monopolization came about through
the formation of the American Medical Association in 1847.
The new strategy was largely the product of one man, Nathan

---

[62] Kaufman, *op. cit.*, pp. 63-75.

Smith Davis, a medical doctor and instructor of pathology in New York, who apparently possessed a remarkable intuitive sense of political organization. The logic of his historically important and sociologically illuminating argument can help clarify the political effects of his strategy. Fortunately, he left an account of his activities for us in two books. One of them, *A History of Medical Education,* is his own description of his strategy, and the analysis presented here will be based on that work.

The idea of a national medical association was not Davis'. As early as 1835, the Medical College of Georgia had called for such a convention, though little came of the proposal. The purpose of such a convention was manifestly the upgrading of educational standards in medicine, but the proposal was reportedly killed by indifference on the part of older Eastern schools.[63] An invitation in 1839 by the Medical Society of the State of New York to all colleges and societies similarly received no response.[64]

The contribution which Davis made was unique and had the most profound long-range consequences for monopolization. It was "the separation of teaching and licensing" by placing licensure functions in state licensing boards appointed by medical societies. The new licensing plan differed from the old by proposing to close alternative portals of entry into the profession; a diploma would no longer be an acceptable alternative to licensure, but a prerequisite. Such a licensing plan had been proposed in 1837 by the medical faculty in Philadelphia, only then the power of licensing review was to have been placed in a practitioner legislature.[65] Davis' contribution was to see the ultimate organizational utility of such a control over diplomas and the necessity of dissociating licensing from apparent practitioner control as a solution to the problem of popular antimonopolistic sentiment.

Davis perceived several organizational problems which

[63] Rosemary Stevens, *American Medicine and the Public Interest* (New Haven: Yale University Press, 1971), pp. 28-29.

[64] *Ibid.,* p. 29.

[65] N. S. Davis, *History of Medical Education and Institutions in the United States, From the First Settlement of the British Colonies to the Year 1850* (Chicago: S. C. Griggs & Co., 1851), p. 194.

could be solved by his strategy. These included the recent proliferation of medical schools and physician with diplomas, the decline in visible functionality of medical societies, and the financial impoverishment of medical societies. These three problems, of course, were closely interrelated.

The inclination of state legislatures to provide medical colleges with charters of incorporation became more relevant after the introduction of general incorporation laws, for these resulted in a rapid increase in the number of medical schools. Davis noted this proliferation (Table 3).

Table 3

Medical Education During the First Half of the Nineteenth Century

Decade	New Medical Schools	Student Total	Graduates	Graduate/ Total Ratio
1810	6	650	100	1 : 6.5
1820	5	964	182	1 : 5.3
1830	8	2125	597	1 : 3.6
1840	11	2800	775	1 : 3.6
1850	13	4500	1300	1 : 3.4

Source: Davis, *Medical Education*, pp. 114–115.

The number of medical students and successful graduates increased even more spectacularly, graduates increasing 1300 percent between 1810 and 1850. In virtually every state, a medical diploma, even under the most restrictive medical licensing laws, was acceptable for entry into the profession. Emphasis on the importance of competition from quackery, then, seems to have been misplaced in light of these figures. Protection of the public against quacks has been a traditional justification for the profession's monopolistic privileges, extending back at least into the Elizabethan period of the Royal College of Physicians of London, and perhaps even further. But it seems that the war on quackery had a somewhat contrived quality in mid-nineteenth-century America, at least from the point of view of the profession's most essential problems of interest pursuit. Though statistical evidence is at best shaky, the proportion of irregular practitioners probably did not exceed 10 percent of all practitioners.

Approximately 2,400 homeopaths practiced in the United States at one time or another between 1835 and 1860, the great majority after 1845. Adding a guess about Eclectic and Physio-Medical strength, there were perhaps 7,000 sectarian practitioners in the 1845-60 period. In the same period there were some 20,000 orthodox medical graduates and about 40,000 orthodox matriculants who never bothered to take degrees. This would give a proportion of one sectarian to 8.50 orthodox physicians.[66]

This figure might have been interpreted at the time as "hordes" of quacks, but it really seems quite small in terms of economic rationality. In retrospect, the leading challenge to the stability of the organized medical societies appears to have come from the explosion in the number of medical schools throughout the country. Competition from irregulars was not nearly as threatening to the interests of the organized profession as was the competition latent in the rapid proliferation of regularly educated physicians.

N.S. Davis attempted to indict the existing system of medical education in terms of built-in incentives for low standards of education. He particularly objected to placing the power of examination into the hands of the same teachers who instructed the examinees and to permitting the examiners to receive payment for each diploma granted.

It is thus seen that every faculty of professors, so far from being disinterested and impartial examiners of their own classes, are under the direct influence of the strongest motive to swell, as far as possible, the list of successful candidates. These motives are nothing less than personal reputation and pecuniary gain, stimulated by the direct competition of rival institutions. Hence, every faculty of professors who resolve themselves into a board of examination, to sit in judgment on the qualifications of their own students, are placed in such a position, that their own personal interests are in direct

[66] Kett, *op. cit.* (n. 20, above), p. 186.

collision with their duty to the whole community, and
their regard for the honor and welfare of the profession
to which they belong.[67]

Davis did not consider, however, that the same sort of
incentives might play a comparable role for the organized
medical profession, only in the direction of restricting the
number of successful candidates. Nor did he consider the
practical possibility of having examiners from different medical schools review the education of graduates. Instead, he
called for the separation of licensing and teaching, that is,
removing the power of entry into the profession from the
hands of academics.

Davis also provided data about the functions of medical
societies. He found that the ratio of diplomas from New York
medical colleges to licenses from state or county medical
societies had decreased from 1:3 in 1820 (38 to "three times
that number") to 1:2 (56:117) in 1830 to 30:1 (246:8) in 1846.[68]
The increasing use of diplomas for entry into the profession,
reinforced by the repeal of medical licensing law penalties,
denied the medical societies one of their most important
functions and justifications for their power and existence:
licensing. Hooker, as has been seen, attempted to resurrect
the war on quackery as the raison d'être of the medical
societies. Davis, however, had a more appropriate idea in
attempting to redefine the function of organized medicine
as the upgrading of standards of medical education. Not only
was it more original, but it lay the foundation for the
domination of medical colleges. He also had the political
sagacity to lay a strategy of indirect domination by calling
for the establishment of licensing boards outside of the
medical societies. The new raison d'être of the medical
societies became the spearheading of the movement to bring
about legislation which would pressure medical schools into
a specific line of development.

The organized profession was also threatened economically
by the decline in numbers of candidates for medical society

[67] N. S. Davis, op. cit., p. 188.
[68] Ibid., p. 116.

licenses, since medical societies were financed through examination fees. According to Davis, this loss of funds resulted
in the neglect of medical society libraries, diminishing interest and attendance at meetings, general indifference on the
part of the profession, the cessation of active existence of
many local societies, and even the repeal of licensing legislation![69]

> So true was this, though state and district medical
> societies had previously been formed in all the eastern
> states—in New York, New Jersey, Delaware, Maryland,
> Mississippi, Alamaba, Tennessee, Ohio, Indiana, and
> Michigan, yet, in 1840, those in Massachusetts and New
> York were almost the only ones that maintained any-
> thing more than a mere nominal existence. And in the
> latter state, out of its sixty counties, not more than 16
> or 17 were represented in the meetings of the state
> society.[70]

Davis' solution consisted in the formation of state boards
of medical examiners and licensing, increasing the length of
medical education, and reviewing the preliminary education
of applicants to medical schools. Preliminary education
would be directly reviewed by the medical societies, thereby
providing a direct veto on the number of students entering
medical schools. Lengthening education would discourage
some students from pursuing this course of education and
might also result in higher quality education. Medical societies were to have a heavy influence on state licensing boards,
thereby affording a final veto on the size of the profession.
Most important, in 1846, a national medical convention,
which resulted in the formation of the American Medical
Asociation, was called for the purpose of investigating the
separation of teaching and licensing. At that time, the
composition of the state boards was proposed as "in fair
proportion of representatives from its state's medical colleges, and the profession at large."[71] Following the AMA's
formation, specifics were proposed: "This board should con-

[69] *Ibid.*, pp. 116-118.
[70] *Ibid.*, pp. 212-213.
[71] *Ibid.*, p. 139.

sist of, at least, seven members, appointed by the state medical society of each state; and, if advisable, also, one additional member, appointed by each regularly incorporated medical college; and the presence of two-thirds should constitute a quorum for the transaction of business."[72]. In this way, as many as six-sevenths of the board members could be representatives of the state medical societies. By these three means, the medical societies might go a long way toward dominating the medical schools, closing the diploma as a simple means of entry into the profession, and laying the infrastructure for the restriction of the size of the medical profession.

The use of state medical licensing boards for indirect domination and monopolization represents a remarkable innovation by Davis. The English self-regulatory tradition in medicine tended to favor the postcolonial Massachusetts arrangement, in which licensing functions were exercised by practitioner organizations. The German tradition in medicine, however, contributed the idea of state licensing superimposed on university examinations. Davis selectively combined the two. The German tradition is noteworthy as an alternative to Davis' formulation. According to the great German surgeon Billroth, a contemporary of Davis, state licensing examinations were given by university faculty members in medicine, whenever they could be induced to leave their studies for this "irksome task." Nonacademic practitioners could have served on these examination boards but for various reasons did not. The German medical schools thus tended to escape practitioner domination, and regulation of the size of the practicing profession tended to come under academic rather than practitioner control. Billroth personally thought the idea of using practitioners to examine candidates for entry into the profession totally irrational because of the inferior intellectual condition of most practitioners, particularly those who could find time to administer examinations.[73] No discussion of the relative merits of academic licensing apparently ever took place in America; Davis'

[72] *Ibid.*, pp. 207-208.
[73] Theodor Billroth, *The Medical Sciences in the German Universities* (New York: The Macmillan Company, 1924), pp. 115-119.

program seems to have diverted attention away from the problem of strengthening medical academics by emphasizing the problems of strengthening the controls of the medical societies over professional affairs.

The significance of these considerations is revealed by Davis' explanation for the formation of the AMA. Davis states that his original intent in proposing the separation of teaching and licensing at an 1844 meeting of the New York State Medical Society was to provide a source of income for the failing medical societies by placing the power of licensing back into the hands of the organized profession.[74] The proposal was discussed further in 1845 in New York, when it led to the call for a national medical convention to be held in 1846. According to Davis, the discussion of this proposal gave rise to the call for the convention.[75] The convention resulted in the formation of the American Medical Association, which held its first meeting in 1847, with Davis as one of its most active secretaries and influential committee members.

The relationship of Davis' strategy to the problem of the restriction of membership in the profession is somewhat clouded by his suggestion that state legislatures finance medical education. Specifically, he proposed that lecture fees be entirely abolished and medical education be made available free to every deserving student.[76] This proposal would at first glance appear opposed to restrictionist tendencies in educational reform, but Davis did not see it that way. He defended this proposal against the charge that "cheapening medical education would only increase the number of those who would crowd into the profession" by arguing that "the numbers should be restricted by adding to the standard of requirements, instead of increasing the exactions on the students' pockets."[77] The point clarifies a great deal. The task he faced was to protect the interests of both organized practitioners and the medical colleges. The former would benefit from upgraded standards by achieving the restriction

[74] N. S. Davis, *op. cit.*, p. 215.
[75] *Ibid.*, p. 196.
[76] *Ibid.*, p. 222.
[77] *Ibid.*, p. 227.

of numbers of practitioners—such, he admits, formed his thought—and the latter need not suffer from restriction if the economic needs of medical schools were met by public financing rather than from private sources.

Davis' proposal for state licensing boards solved the organizational problems which the organized profession faced. The rapid proliferation of medical schools and graduates might be checked by the imposition of rigidly upgraded standards, watched over by the licensing boards. The function of the medical societies would be to upgrade standards and to supply official definition of the profession's boundaries and composition by having representatives of the state medical societies man the boards. Charges of monopoly directed at the medical societies might be avoided by placing the restrictive powers of licensing in state boards. Moreover, the economic needs of the medical societies would be served by providing the societies with an organizational basis for pushing the interests of practitioners, giving them drawing power for dues and contributions from members.

Implementation of Davis' proposals, however, was not yet in sight. Legislatures in most states did not establish state medical licensing boards for yet another half-century and medical schools were not about to abandon a relatively advantageous situation merely to preserve the medical societies. Some schools tried changing the length of curriculum and various means of upgrading the quality of the curriculum, and a few schools reduced their tuition fees, ostensibly in keeping with the AMA's recommendations. Yet, in general, the medical schools ignored the AMA's attempt to coordinate them: ". . . we are most gravely told by each college, that it is ready to comply with the recommendation so soon as all the other colleges shall do the same; and, at the end of three years, with very few exceptions, each is still waiting for all the others."[78] Fundamentally, the proposal to upgrade educational standards by regulating entry into the profession at multiple points along the educational process did not take into account the need to regulate education. Preliminary education was still provided by individual preceptor-practi-

[78] *Ibid.*, p. 200.

tioners of varying quality, and lengthening already poor
courses did not meet the problem. Without state aid to
medical schools, much as Davis anticipated, the medical
schools would not abandon their reliance on student fees
and large enrollments.

On a more general level, the medical colleges had no
interest in complying with the de facto instructions of the
organized practitioners. And without state licensing boards,
the diploma still remained the portal of entry into the
profession.[79] In time, professional teaching in the colleges
by academics would replace the system of apprenticeship
for preliminary education, and state licensing boards would
be instituted, leaving the other two problems of medical
school financing and the quality of medical teaching up to
the medical schools and the medical societies, respectively.
For the time being, however, the AMA's program remained
unfulfilled until a more hospitable institutional soil developed in the state legislatures.

The period of antitrust legislation (post-1890)

The three earlier periods in this chapter have dealt with
the general problem of the consequences of the relative
failure of medical societies to monopolize the practice of
medicine; this fourth period will consider the relatively
successful monopolistic accomplishments of American organized medicine. Between 1880 and 1900, the organized
medical profession succeeded in having state licensing boards,
dominated in whole or in part by representatives of the
state medical societies, established in every state. This ac-
complishment, one might note, was in accordance with N.S.
Davis' earlier plans. The first state board for medical licensing was established under medical society control during the
1870's in Texas, but was virtually "inoperative, as but few
boards are organized, and about most that any of them do
is license non-graduates."[80] Many of these boards of the 1870's
functioned as little more than registration boards, where
physicians might register their medical society licenses or

---

[79] Corner, op. cit. (n. 35, above), p. 101.
[80] Fitz, "Legislative Control," p. 612.

medical college diplomas. Nonetheless laws requiring state boards for medical licensing were passed at an accelerated rate during the 1880's and 1890's (Table 4). By 1898, all states and territories of the United States except for Alaska had medical licensing boards.[81]

Table 4

Medical Practice Restriction Acts in the United States

Date of Passage	State of Passage
1880	Vermont
1882	Georgia, Rhode Island
1883	Maine, Michigan, North Carolina
1884	New Mexico
1885	Indiana
1886	Iowa
1887	California, Idaho, Minnesota, Virginia, Wisconsin, Wyoming
1888	Tennessee
1889	Delaware, Kansas, Missouri, Montana, Oregon
1890	New Jersey, North Dakota, Ohio, South Carolina, Washington
1891	Colorado, Nebraska, West Virginia
1892	Florida, Maryland, Mississippi, Utah
1893	Arkansas, Arizona, Connecticut, Kentucky, New York, Oklahoma, Pennsylvania, South Dakota

Source: Fitz, *op. cit.*, p. 613.

Yet these institutional changes are problematic in light of earlier periods in American medical history. The AMA had officially proposed such an arrangement as early as 1847; a prototypical model for such legislation had existed in Maryland during the first four decades of the nineteenth century. So, if Davis' estimation of the Maryland experience had been that they were "simple and effectual laws," why was there then a delay of some thirty to fifty years before state legislatures consented to pass this sort of legislation? Furthermore, why was this monopolistic legislation paradoxically passed during the height of the antitrust movement in America? The Sherman Act had been passed in 1890, when public opinion was reportedly running strongly against mon-

[81] Shryock, *op. cit.* (n. 33, above), pp. 54-55.

opolies and trusts.[82] It seems remarkable that such an appreciable degree of monopolistic control over the size of the profession could have been acquired at a time of intense nation-wide antimonopolistic feeling.

While the first part of this chapter has tried to explain how antimonopolistic ideologies inhibited the institutionalization of the medical profession as a self-regulating group during the first part of the nineteenth century, the remainder will try to explain why antimonopolistic ideologies did not inhibit monopolization during the last part of the century. This does not mean that there was no opposition to medical monopolization. As will be seen, specific charges of "medical monopoly" were made against the organized profession. These forces, however, were not able to gather sufficient strength to prevent monopolization.

One might think that the change in the receptivity of state legislatures to the idea of medical licensing was simply a result of increasing scientific competence in medicine; such, however, might not have been the case. The most productive advances in medicine were not to come until the twentieth century. The scientific method, in fact, had not entered American medicine until the 1860's. Orthodox medicine was still very much in a period of therapeutic nihilism, engaged in examining traditional practices with controlled studies for evidence of efficacy, at the time when the medical licensing laws were passed. The competence of the medical profession was probably not very convincing, even in the eyes of contemporary legislators; many states of the period passed licensing legislation which permitted irregular practitioners to practice, as long as they could pass a qualifying examination. For several decades many physicians had taken Hooker's position and insisted that the public was capable of selecting competent physicians only on the basis of professional reputation and ethical standing and that legislation was not necessary. In short, one cannot simply say that obvious advantages for the public of medical practice laws resulted in their passage.

Even if a strong case had been built for the public advan-

[82] William Letwin, *Law and Economic Policy in America: The Evolution of the Sherman Antitrust Act* (New York: Random House, 1965), pp. 54-59.

tages of such laws, the reasons for the receptivity of legislators to these proposals would still not be clear. What one
also needs to understand is the political significance of these
laws to explain why they were passed. The public interest
notwithstanding, strong political forces opposed to such
changes could have prevented the passage of legislation.
From the positive side, one would like to know which particular interests of legislators resulted in their passing this
legislation. Although some plausible interpretation in terms
of the public interest was probably necessary for the passage
of medical practice laws, it was probably not sufficient. It
is also important to know the constellation of interests in
which these changes occurred, and particularly the reasons
for which charges of monopoly were disregarded.

Some clues are available about the interest context in
which medical legislation was passed, but a definitive investigation still remains to be done. Nonetheless, certain statements can be made about the social context of the origin
of these laws. First, there was little or no compatibility between professional monopolization and ruling-class ideologies favoring corporate monopolization. In defense of monopolization in terms of the public interest, the ideologies of
the large corporate monopolies stressed the general social
utility and inevitability of the rise of monopolies in terms
of efficiency, scale of production, and market stabilization.[83]
They were laissez faire ideologies to the extent that they
opposed government action against the formation and operation of monopolies, and prided themselves on having achieved
economic success without apparent aid from the state (even
if such were not the case in reality). On none of these counts
could the medical profession claim continuity. The profession
did not attribute its social utility to its largeness or stabilizing
effects on the market or make any claims in terms of
economic consequences. Instead of seeing its effectiveness
and utility as inevitable, an outcome of "natural" competitive forces in the market, it stressed the importance of
regulating market forces in the sphere of medicine to protect
the consumer from fraudulent practitioners. Moreover, it was

[83] William Lee Baldwin, *Antitrust and the Changing Corporation* (Durham, N.C.:
Duke University Press, 1961), pp. 7-9.

committed to state intervention in behalf of the public;
licensure did, after all, make the profession a legally privileged group.

This last point contains an important insight: the monopoly of the medical profession has been of a different type
than that of the corporate monopolies of the late nineteenth
century—a legally privileged group rather than a market-
derived monopoly. Thus, the medical profession was not able
to take advantage of ruling-class monopolistic ideologies
during this period as it had during the age of federalism.
Its type of monopolization did not fit as a subtype of
corporate monopolization or ride in with the success of that
type of monopolization. Therefore, one must look elsewhere
to explain the successful monopolization of the profession.

The most plausible source for an explanation of the rise
of the medical profession and of the professions in general
in the United States lies in the political conflict between
local and national economic interests. This judgment rests
on three considerations. First, at the turn of the century
in America, there was a burst of state legislation in favor
of local combinations in restraint of trade for independent
retailers, small town producers, and individual professional
men. This legislation was designed to counteract the economic encroachment of national corporations which had
developed new means of distribution that left local businessmen at an economic disadvantage. In effect, this legislation
stabilized the local economy, in the name of the local public
interest, by providing legal protections in the form of monopolistic rights for local businessmen and legal obstacles for
outside business interests. Much of the legislation, however,
was clearly directed toward eliminating competition from
below—long training periods, examinations, and fees for licensing, all of which were required in a wide variety of
occupations, including plumbers, barbers, and retail dealers,
as well as the learned professions. In many states a residency
period was required as well. These laws protected the economic interests of local business against competitors from
both above and below. Attacks by competitors from below
were prevented by laws blocking the dissipation of local

concentrations of economic power; attacks by competitors from above were prevented by ideological attacks on national corporate business practices. Fear of local competition resulted in a variety of licensing devices to discourage would-be entrants by demanding more than mere competence.[84]

> Through these varying statutes and ordinances, the police powers of the states are being manipulated by pressure groups of small businessmen to bulwark their economic status with legislative monopoly. The suppressed competitor has no effective weapon. He has attacked such monopolies in the courts with arguments based on the Fourteenth Amendment. But for the most part, he has failed. Courts are not traditionally empowered to look behind the ostensible purpose of such legislation to its true designs. If a statute purports to meet a public need and the measures are related to the stated purposes in the slightest degree, the courts have in this field, perhaps more than elsewhere, refrained from questioning the opinion of the legislatures.[85]

There is some evidence, too, of the frequent use of "corporate medicine" during this period, particularly in the Far West where industrial companies not uncommonly hired doctors on salary to provide care for workers. These corporate employers threatened the local practitioners in two senses: by drawing away patients, and by posing the possibility that practitioners organized into groups with the advantage of corporate efficiency and resources would lower fees and the cost of care and thereby simply outcompete local practitioners.

The second consideration, indeed, was the introduction of national corporate business into American communities with consequent economic disruption and tendencies toward social disintegration of these communities.[86] Even though

[84] Lloyd N. Cutler and Staff, "The Legislative Monopolies Achieved by Small Business," *Yale Law Journal* 48 (March 1939), pp. 851-856.

[85] *Ibid.*, pp. 857-858.

[86] Robert H. Wiebe, *The Search for Order: 1877-1920* (New York: Hill and Wang, 1967), pp. 45-49.

medical practitioners were by no means as hard hit as other businessmen, they were able to ride with popular feeling against corporations, expressed in the belief that national economic competition would have to be fought with local business monopolies.

Third, the Sherman Act is now conceded by social historians to have been passed in behalf of local business interests, who opposed the unrestrained competitive monopolization of the national corporations.[87] Typical targets of sentiment against monopoly included the railroad corporations, giant wheat farms ("the land monopoly"), and " 'monster business establishments, owned by private individuals, of which the Standard Oil Company is the best known type.' "[88] The Sherman Act tended to attack specifically national corporations, since it was limited to corporations engaged in interstate commerce, and local monopolies usually did not qualify on this count. State antitrust laws were also passed but were simply not used against local business interests; as of 1939, at least, no cases had been found where monopolistic licensing laws had been successfully attacked as violations of antitrust law.[89]

The prohibition of national monopolies and the encouragement of local monopolies were perfectly consistent actions in terms of protecting local interests, though indeed not philosophically consistent. In the case of medicine, state licensing laws for the medical profession, as for other local businesses and occupational groups, were upheld or left unchallenged by state authorities and the courts, adding these businesses to the fight against new organizational trends in the nation. In so doing, medical licensure became integrated into the emerging struggle against bureaucratization of American life, the leading symbol of which was the corporation:

> Professional men deny that they engage in "trade" or in restraints of trade. But the professions have their own pattern for pegging the *status quo* with a traditional

[87] *Ibid.*, pp. 52-53; Cutler, *op. cit.*, p. 858.
[88] Letwin, *op. cit.*, pp. 68-69.
[89] Cutler, "Legislative Monopolies," p. 858.

price level. Contemporary investigation by the Department of Justice reveals the pressure exerted by the Medical Association of the District of Columbia in opposition to group health plans. Necessarily subject to comparable scrutiny must be the legal doctrines that have so long prohibited corporate practice in all the professions. It is apparent that here, too, is protection of a monopoly of a traditional method and the price fixing implicit in a customary basis for the reckoning of fees. The opponent in the fight is the corporation which would bring into the professions a new method of distributing services and satisfy a demand for lower professional prices. Chief legal weapon of the individualists is the prohibition of "corporate practice" either expressed in statute and years of dicta, or implicit in a legalistic interpretation of the words of a statute limiting practice to "licensed persons," a status which a corporate person cannot attain. On the social level vigorous arguments are made that by dividing loyalties corporate practice impairs the intimate personal relationship which is fundamental to the practice of the professions, and that commercialization is necessarily accompanied by a collapse of ethics.[90]

Even with the advantage of a favorable constellation of interests, the organized medical profession had to answer charges of monopoly. For example in Massachusetts during the 1890's, the monopolization efforts of the local organized medical profession were attacked by the National Constitutional Liberty League of Boston, a group headed by a medical doctor, J. Rhodes Buchanan. Proposed licensing laws were said to be restraints of liberty on the part of both patient and physician and were condemned as leading to the creation of "class legislation" in the form of a medical monopoly. The President of the Massachusetts Medical Society responded by denying that such laws would constitute monopolization. "It does not create a monopoly," he argued, "since it does not limit the practice of medicine to any

[90] *Ibid.*, pp. 851-852.

particular sect or school. Any person can still become a physician by taking the necessary steps to secure a proper preparation for an occupation which is generally conceded to be one of great responsibility, and one demanding a various training. What is open to all is no monopoly."[91] In other words, by denying that the licensing laws provided a monopoly to only a particular group on the basis of group membership, he evaded the relationship of licensing laws to the restraint of trade, a different meaning of monopoly. The logic of his argument was that permitting practice to only those who could demonstrate competence was not inherently restrictive, for everyone was free to acquire competence.

There was some plausibility to this argument, for licensing laws, instituted alone, constitute an imperfect mechanism of monopolization. Upgrading standards to restrict membership in the medical profession has been a fundamental strategy for monopolization, but quite evidently that alone is not a very stable strategy. The possibility that medical colleges might be able to turn out increasing numbers of students capable of passing the licensing examinations always remains. The organized profession, unlike medical schools, has no set number of places in the profession to fill and no fixed membership. The tactic of the organized profession has been to discourage membership by increasing obstacles to entry. There is, then, a tension between the profession's tendency to set standards high enough to restrict membership and the medical schools' tendency to improve education to get over the hurdles. The result is a built-in inflation of standards where, as medical education improves, the standards for entry become stricter.

The organized profession has dealt with this problem of indirect control over the size of the profession by supplementary devices. Elton Rayack has emphasized the monopolistic significance of restricting the number of medical schools and the establishment of a system of medical school accreditation.[92] The historical record, indeed, is consistent with the restrictive character of particular AMA policies. Following

[91] Fitz, "Legislative Control," p. 583.
[92] Rayack, *op. cit.* (n. 7, above), pp. 66-72.

the publication of the Flexner Report in 1910, which was an investigation of the condition of medical schools by the Carnegie Foundation, the AMA's Council on Medical Education began to grade schools on an A or B basis. Faced by such a situation, these schools might have been expected to have either improved standards or closed down. Most, in fact virtually all, chose the latter: the number of schools dropped from 154 in 1904 to 80 (including five sectarian colleges) in 1928 and to 66 in 1933. This final number corresponds very closely with the ratings of 1913: 24 schools had been rated A+, 39 as A, and physicians to population dropped from 1 : 600 in 1900 to 1 : 763 in 1938.[93]

Even if medical licensing laws were not inherently restrictive, clearly they have been used restrictively. This observation raises the question of the relationship of the extant medical profession in America to antitrust legislation. My explanation for the origin of medical legislation during the antitrust period still does not fully account for the persistence of this legislation in the face of antitrust suits by the government and private parties.

The fact that the medical profession has not been broken up, as have certain giant corporations, does not mean that it is not open for prosecution under the antitrust laws. One needs to inquire, then, into the legal vulnerability of the American medical profession in order to ascertain whether the problem of the profession's persistence is a real one. This task is simplified by the 1943 Supreme Court case of the American Medical Association versus the United States. A complaint was brought by the United States Justice Department against the Medical Society of the District of Columbia after the expulsion of physicians who had agreed to participate in the Group Health Association (GHA), a cooperative designed to provide low-cost medical services to members. Expulsion from the medical society in this case brought denial of hospital privileges for GHA physicians, because of the influence of the medical society over hospital staffing policies. The medical society also circulated a "white list"

[93] Shryock, op. cit. (n. 33, above), 62-64.

of approved physicians and organizations to society members and Washington hospitals, omitting GHA and thereby preventing consultations.[94] The AMA and Medical Society of the District of Columbia were found guilty of conspiracy to engage in restraint of trade.

Similar actions have been brought by health service organizations and private physicians against lower-level medical societies which have attempted to eliminate internal competition by expulsion of member physicians or by refusal of membership to otherwise qualified physicians.[95] Unfortunately, these instances of legal action against professional control mechanisms obscure the more fundamental problem of the legal status of licensure as a method for the restraint of trade.

(The following arguments might be made to explain why the medical profession is not legally open to prosecution for monopolization.) First, one might claim that the medical profession is not subject to federal prosecution, since it does not engage in interstate commerce to any appreciable degree.) Fundamentally, such seems to be the case; but federal prosecution is possible in one specific case, and prosecution by other authorities might be possible. The Sherman Act specifically applies to all trade activities within the District of Columbia, since it is not a state. This is why the case of the AMA versus the United States was initiated in the District of Columbia, where engaging in interstate commerce is not necessary for prosecution. Also, nearly every state possesses antitrust legislation similar to the Sherman Act. Theoretically, at least, the medical profession could be prosecuted state by state, perhaps led by the efforts of the Justice Department in Washington against the District of Columbia's profession.

Second, there is the argument that the medical profession is a profession and not a trade, and therefore cannot be convicted of engaging in restraint of trade. In the 1943 case of AMA versus the United States, however, the medical

[94] Hyde, "Power, Purpose, and Politics," pp. 990-991.
[95] Richard A. Posner, et al., "Judicially Compelled Admission to Medical Societies: The Falcone Case," *Harvard Law Review* 75 (1962), pp. 1186-1198.

profession was deemed a trade by the Supreme Court,
thereby reversing an earlier district court decision, because
the "'calling or occupation of ... defendents ... [is] ...
immaterial if the purpose and effect of their conspiracy was
such obstruction and restraint.'"[96]

Third, there is the argument that learned professions are
exempted from antitrust legislation, as are certain other
organizations. The 1943 action, however, also calls this argument into question. In federal antitrust legislation, the three
main exemptions consist of labor unions, public utilities, and
agricultural cooperatives. Of these, labor unions are permitted under section six of the 1914 Clayton Act to promote
the interests of their members, regardless of effects upon
business competition. Labor unions are only restricted from
entering into collusive agreements with business employers
to circumvent the intention of the antitrust laws. Public
utilities, on the other hand, are viewed as unavoidable or
practical monopolies, which are directly regulated by federal
agencies and therefore exempted. Agricultural cooperatives
are constrained from price enhancing, through the regulatory
powers of the Secretary of Agriculture. In general, the
problem of the value of certain monopolies for the public
interest is resolved by either requiring regulatory control or
permitting monopolization only to those in an obviously
disadvantageous position of power with respect to their
employers. The legal justification for the exemption of labor
unions is that "the labor of a human being is not a commodity
or article of commerce."[97] While one might therefore think
that, for legal purposes, medical services could be considered
labor and the organized medical profession a labor union,
the 1943 ruling that medical practice is a trade excludes it
from the protection of labor union exemption. Organized
medicine's ideological claims to be of benefit for the public
as a service organization would also tend to classify it with
public utility monopolies rather than with unions, yet it is

[96] Miriam Lashley, et al., "Group Health Plans: Some Legal and Economic
Aspects," *Yale Law Journal* 53 (1943), p. 180.
[97] A. D. Neale, *The Antitrust Laws of the United States of America: A Study
of Competition Enforced by Law* (Cambridge: At the University Press, 1962), pp.
5-11.

a public utility without evidence of external regulation.

The fourth argument is that the medical profession, when all is said and done, is a desirable monopoly from the standpoint of society and therefore should be permitted. While such may indeed be the case, judicial opinion currently does not accept such arguments. "Indeed, it may be said that every restrictive practice that significantly impairs competition is illegal *per se* in modern antitrust, since evidence challenging the desirability of unimpaired competition is scarcely ever admissible."[98] Recent decisions that specific business practices are not illegal per se have not referred to consequences for the public interest; they simply mean that impairment of competition is illegal per se, even if it should further the public interest. Therefore, within the legal philosophy of contemporary antitrust interpretations, the public advantages of medical legislation and monopolistic practices do not excuse the profession from prosecution. At least in legal theory, the American medical profession might be prosecuted for engaging in restraint of trade on the basis of having used licensing laws to restrict the size of the profession.

Failure to prosecute the medical profession has not stemmed from overwhelming legal difficulties. Even though difficult to specify, probably the most important forces in favor of the profession's continued monopolization have been political. Certainly, no significant political force has congealed to oppose the profession's monopolization. One wonders what part the monopolization interests of lawyers, another profession, have played in the legal profession's disinclination to take on the organized medical profession; to expect the legal profession to attack its own basis for interest pursuit does seem politically unrealistic. Yet legal codes notwithstanding, the belief that some monopolies are socially desirable persists, in favor of the profession's monopolization. Perhaps the personal experiences of lawyers with physicians have tended to predispose them favorably to the profession's claims to be acting in behalf of the public interest. Certainly licensing laws which upgrade standards

[98] *Ibid.*, p. 21.

for physicians benefit certain social groups, specifically those which can best afford high physician fees and auxiliary costs, even if these laws result in a restricted membership and lack of care for the less wealthy. A group with monopolistic tendencies can exist because it satisfactorily meets the needs or interests of the groups that rule society—in the case of America, of the wealthier middle class and the upper classes, which include lawyers and the controllers of local policies. Obviously, this question has not yet been fully investigated or answered, and the political as well as legal attitudes of lawyers toward the medical profession seem to be an important and appropriate area for future investigation.

In summary, it appears that the successful monopolization efforts of the American medical profession during an age of antitrust legislation can be explained in terms of the favorable political interest constellation of that period. This constellation provided certain local business groups with monopolistic advantages which they might otherwise never have acquired had not local communities been threatened with progressive external control by national corporate interests. Competition between local and national economic interests has persisted to the present day, but there is little evidence that the local control gained by the medical profession has yet been substantially reduced by national forces. It is to this question of the profession's stabilization of its position within a changing constellation of forces that this study now turns.

The role of the American Medical Association

Much has already been said about the origins of the AMA and its role in formulating an indirect monopolization strategy which has served as the basis for contemporary medical institutions in America. It is enlightening to go beyond this aspect and examine the role of the AMA within the interest constellation of successful licensing legislation. When one reads the essays by Milton Friedman and the editors of the *Yale Law Journal* on the medical profession as a monopoly, an impression is gained that the state medical societies are but puppet extensions or arms of the central control agency

of the AMA. Against this oligarchical imagery appears contradictory evidence of apparently sincere support of the AMA
by the vast majority of rank-and-file member practitioners.[99]
There are also claims by the AMA of representation of the
interests of the medical profession on a local level, that is,
that it is a relatively democratic body which cannot force
local societies to accede to demands.

In light of the interest constellation in the United States,
the AMA's own statements about its political nature should
be taken more seriously than they have been by social
scientists. The answer to the question of *cui bono* suggests
why. Medical licensure brought the state medical societies
back to life, so to speak. They had found a new public service
function to legitimize their power and secured various degrees
of legal protection. Membership increased, and attention
began to turn toward continuing the protection of recent
accomplishments on a state level against events on the
national scene. The AMA was reorganized in 1901, by and
large excluding nonpractitioners and lay groups from membership, and establishing a new system of internal government which would facilitate more rapid policy making.[100] The
challenge then was to prevent bureaucratic changes in the
federal government and private business enterprise from
undoing what had been gained. Membership in the AMA
jumped from 8400 in 1900 to over 70,000 by 1910.[101] The AMA
immediately issued a model plan for the organization of state
and county medical societies,[102] which was followed by many
societies. Yet it made no attempts to regulate the practice
of medicine; indeed the AMA devoted the greatest part of
its effort to either bringing about new legislation more
favorable to the interests of the local medical profession or
blocking the development of new modes of medical care
delivery, particularly by private and public national forces.
In this perspective, the AMA emerges, despite its leader-

[99] Oliver Garceau, *The Political Life of the American Medical Association* (Hamden, Connecticut: Archon Books, 1961 [1941]), pp. 136-137.
[100] James G. Burrow, *AMA: Voice of American Medicine* (Baltimore: Johns
Hopkins Press, 1963), pp. 27-33.
[101] Wiebe, *op. cit.* (n. 86, above), p. 115.
[102] Burrow, *op. cit.*, pp. 36-44.

ship role in providing organizational models and tools for
state medical societies, as the political arm of the state
medical societies against national developments. Domination
of the AMA over state societies seems to be more or less
limited to that necessary to prevent interstate competition.
It has indeed prepared policy stands which have been adopted
by state societies, but these stands were devised by representatives of the state societies, sitting on the Board of
Trustees and in the House of Delegates of the AMA. Until
recently, no substantial political group within the AMA has
yet successfully arisen to oppose AMA interests over those
of the state societies; there are, however, as will be discussed
in the following chapter, AMA reformers who would like
to restructure the organization of the AMA in order to
mobilize physicians in behalf of national medical policies set
by the AMA or through a coopted health institute.

Recapitulation

In this chapter, it has been found that the American
medical profession has followed an indirect and diffuse type
of monopolization strategy compared to that of the Royal
College of Physicians of London. In looking into the history
of the profession, one finds that colonial attempts to institute
RCP-type legal privileges failed because of either preexisting
RCP privileges or the interest of local administrators in
demonstrating their own autonomy vis-à-vis England by
issuing licenses. After the Revolution, the medical profession
won varying degrees of control over licensing, but these
licenses had little capacity for restricting competition. They
frequently lacked sanctions, gave the profession an unfavorable public reputation for monopolistic persecution of unlicensed practitioners, were rarely enforced by the courts, and
did not in any event close alternative portals of entry into
the profession.

The advent of general incorporation legislation in the early
nineteenth century resulted in a proliferation of medical
schools, and the number of orthodox practitioners swelled.
The medical societies issued fewer licenses, since medical
degrees were preferred permits of entry into the profession,

and instead abandoned licensing in favor of substituting state licenses for medical school diplomas as the sole legal privilege to practice. Despite antitrust legislation and popular opinion against monopolies, state boards were established at the end of the nineteenth century and were legally dominated by filling at least a majority of each board with representatives of the state medical societies. Medical school admissions were curtailed by spiraling accreditation standards for licensing and by medical education laws requiring certain types of training preparation. In this instance, antimonopolistic ideologies were not politically decisive because of the coincidence of the monopolistic interests of practitioners with the monopolistic interests of local business elites—the same interest groups which ironically pushed for antitrust legislation.

This chapter has tried to explain the differential success of the profession's monopolistic behavior in terms of the interest constellation between the profession and politically significant groups. Not until the American profession found itself in a politically favorable position because of changing conditions of competition was it able to use licensing for monopolization with any appreciable effect. The theoretical perspective has changed, however, in this chapter. Previously, ethics and licensure were seen as constituents of an interest group's monopolization strategy. Several instances of apparent demonopolization, placed in the context of the position of the profession with respect to other groups, were interpreted as instances of indirect monopolization created in response to political pressures. This shifted the unit of analysis from the interest group to society as a posited whole. Instead of trying to grasp merely the organized profession's monopolization strategy, one should consider the interactive effects of society's receptivity to the profession's behavior. This chapter has not merely noted the compatibility of the profession's ideologies with ruling-class ideologies, as in the English chapter; it has also considered the compatibility of the profession's interests with ruling-class interests.

In following Weber's indications and examining the conditions of social receptivity to monopolization, one finds that social receptivity applies in both negative and positive senses. Successful monopolization can be explained by the failure of antimonopolistic forces to prevent the process from occurring. This negative explanation should be considered on several levels. First, there is the selective nature of antimonopoly movements due to variation in definitions of monopoly. Antimonopolistic movements as well as monopolies have their wider political uses by ruling groups, and these uses should be understood in order to explain why certain targets are selected for antimonopolistic action. Antimonopolistic movements are typically directed primarily at nonmedical monopolists, and medicine has become relevant only as a subclass of more general phenomena. So, while under one social definition of monopoly the medical profession's monopolization tactics may run into opposition, under another definition they may not gain much attention. Second, even in the face of constant antimonopolistic forces, the monopolistic tactics of the medical profession have by no means remained constant. Whenever the selective nature of antimonopolistic ideologies has not let the medical profession go unmolested, the profession has searched for loopholes in the structure of the ideology. It has adopted tactics and ideologies which exempt it from the terms of the ideology. Third, even though the terms of an antimonopolistic ideology may still apply to the medical profession, political forces necessary to oppose the medical profession may not congeal. This type of phenomenon is apparently commonplace in antitrust cases, where the law may forbid certain practices but legal action is not taken against offenders on account of mitigating or expedient reasons or simply insufficient political interest. Fourth, the political strength of groups interested in pushing antimonopolistic ideologies may not be sufficient to depose the profession from its advantageous position, because of countervailing political groups in society. The courts, for instance, may not interpret antimonopolistic laws in the same manner as antitrust lawyers might.

The question of antimonopolistic movements is most relevant to the issue of society's receptivity to the form of the organization of the profession. Another issue which should be mentioned is society's receptivity to the consequences of the profession's organization. The more recent politics of consumer demand for services, for instance, have tended to judge the profession in terms of its capacity to meet those demands, rather than the formal character of its organization. Occasionally, certain monopolistic features of the organized profession have come under attack because of their apparent role as obstacles to meeting those demands, but this type of social constraint is different from a wholesale attack on monopolization per se.

Positively, there have been the political uses of monopolies by groups other than the interest group. The use of royal monopolies by the English Stuarts for mercantilist purposes of financing state building is a classic example of how this might work.[103] Monopolies may come into existence out of their utility for some group other than the interest group and may persist for similar reasons. As has been demonstrated this particular positive explanation for mercantilist monopolization has not exactly applied to the American medical profession: unlike the mercantilist monopolies, the profession's profits from monopolization have not been shared with outsiders. Yet, ultimately, one would wish some type of positive explanation for why legal privileges were extended to the medical profession. Apparently, the conversion of medical services into a valued reward for the success of a particular social class explains the interest that powerful groups in American society have had in permitting the profession's monopolization. Hence, one finds the interests of specific groups—particularly ruling groups—and not the public interest most informative. Explanations in terms of the public interest simply tend to be excessively nonspecific, especially in light of the differential distribution of the benefits of medical care. Not all groups which compose society have benefited from the monopolization of medical services, and this very condition helps explain better why monopolization has occurred.

[103] Max Weber, *Economy and Society: An Outline of Interpretive Sociology*, eds. Guenther Roth and Claus Wittich, 3 vols. (New York: Bedminster Press, 1968), p. 1098.

CHAPTER SIX

American Medical Reform
and Monopolization

So far, this discussion of the way in which the English and American medical professions pursued monopolization has shown how both emerged from a common monopolization strategy, that of the Royal College of Physicians, but diverged according to political circumstance. This chapter will deal with how the AMA has traditionally applied its legal privileges in behalf of monopolization and will then examine a current proposal for reorganizing the AMA in an ostensibly less monopolistic direction. As before, the monopolistic consequences of these antimonopolistic reforms will be investigated, to see if perhaps the AMA is creating a new type of monopolistic strategy which is in fact more monopolistic than the old one. This chapter will also expand knowledge of the political conditions of monopolization, trying to look beyond antimonopolistic ideologies for other major types of constraints on monopolization. Finally, it will elucidate the AMA's failure to adopt these reforms, thereby making for a more comprehensive theory, and will argue that the potential for more effective monopolization need not lead to pursuit of that potential.

The AMA's traditional monopolization strategy

The end of the last chapter discussed the role of the AMA as a political arm of the interests of the state medical societies. It is of interest, now, why and how the AMA has opposed in the past a variety of national forces which have proposed altering the organization of the practice of medicine. "Why" in this context refers not to the profession's manifest justifications for opposition but to the relationship of these objections to the profession's interest position, and as such, to the profession's monopolization pattern. What haa the AMA's apparent monopolization strategy been for dealing with intrusive national groups?

One AMA tactic has been the opposition of "bureaucratic" types of organization. When it has talked of bureaucracy, it has referred to three interest-relevant phenomena, singly or in combination: contract practice, prepaid plans, and group practice. In different ways, these forms of organization have threatened the monopolization interests of the conventional medical profession. In speaking of "organized practice" or "organized practitioners," then, I refer to these alternative forms of organization of physicians. All other references to "organized medicine" and the "organized profession" are synonymous with interest-group organizations like the medical societies and the AMA. Therefore, I will discuss how "organized practice" has been opposed by the "organized profession."

How the use of contract practice could threaten the profession's collective economic interests is suggested by John Duffy's review of the organized medical profession's experience in Louisiana with the "contract system." Since colonial days, physicians had contracted on an annual salary basis with plantation owners to care for their families and slaves. As the supply of physicians gradually increased, however, contract practice became more attractive as a source of patients and income. "Hence, when the New Orleans Medical Protective Association was organized in June of 1875, it expressed strong disapproval of the contract practice 'as tending toward the demoralization and degradation of the profession of medicine, and ruinous to the financial welfare of us all.' "[1] By 1888, it was estimated by the medical

---

[1] John Duffy, ed., *History of Medicine in Louisiana*, 2 vols. (Louisiana State University Press, 1962), vol. II, p. 399.

society journal that four-fifths of the New Orleans population belonged to benevolent societies which provided services on a contract basis. Competition among physicians for employment resulted in underbidding to a point where one physician "offered medical care for as little as forty cents per member."[2] A questionnaire the following year revealed that 41 percent of New Orleans registered physicians engaged in contract practice. Apparently, this competition for positions tended to impoverish the profession as a whole, "and this impoverishment only served to perpetuate the system," presumably by reducing the market for services provided by independent physicians.

Clearly, the threat posed by contract practice was that salaried service in the presence of a net surplus of physicians in the market could be used to drive down the incomes of physicians. Those who charged fees were also pressured into lowering their income in order not to lose their patients to the less expensive contract service plans. In a general way, contract practice represented one way in which organized practitioners could activate economic competition among individual practitioners, and thereby break down efforts toward monopolization.

Prepaid plans, in which prospective patients shared the financial risk of health care by creating a fund to guarantee services for subscribers in times of illness, threatened individual practitioners with increased competition from organized practitioners in a different respect. By combining the costs of medical services with other health care costs, such as hospitalization, diagnostic and therapeutic work, and auxiliary personnel salaries, the prepaid plans were able to offer services to patients at a lower price without necessarily underpaying member physicians. While prepaid plans did not threaten to decrease the profession's income, they threatened independent practitioners with loss of patients and thereby loss of income. Not surprisingly, the AMA opposed prepaid plans which reimbursed only certain physicians in the community.[3]

[2] *Ibid.*, p. 400.
[3] David R. Hyde and Staff, "The American Medical Association: Power, Purpose, and Politics in Organized Medicine," *Yale Law Journal* 63 (May 1954), p. 987.

Group practice was also opposed because it led to increased competition among physicians. During the 1930's, it was disparaged as unethical, but in recent years it has been tolerated by organized medicine unless flat-fee prepayment has been employed.[4] Group practice entailed the cooperative ownership and use of offices and equipment by a group of physicians. Its apparent health benefit for the public represented a threat to economic interests for certain practitioners, however, by promising to reduce the price of health through the reduction of office-operation costs by sharing test equipment, space, and a secretarial staff. For unorganized practitioners, group practice represented a threat by also drawing away patients.

A fourth phenomenon, "corporate practice," apparently combines the previous three. It is a prepaid group practice plan, which reimburses member physicians on the basis of salaries or capitation fees. The presence of lay sponsorship made corporate practice particularly threatening by increasing the probability of orgainzed competition. Laymen were not subject to professional ethical injunctions against price competition, and were less likely to support the profession's tendencies toward fee fixing.

One can readily understand the organized profession's opposition to these forms of "bureaucracy." The organized profession's monopolistic strategy was constructed on the assumption that practitioners would continue to work as individuals, and that all competition would occur among independent practitioners. Simple fee fixing through a traditional scale of fees for services sufficed to eliminate such competition, as long as physicians did not try to undercut one another. Bureaucratization, as it was perceived, threatened to provide organized practitioners with an economic advantage in the market relative to independent practitioners. Organized medicine, (i.e., the medical societies) chose to speak for the interests of independent practitioners.

Within this context, the idealization of the individual practitioner, a problematic ideal, can be clarified. Service ideologies call for a certain measure of evaluation and criti-

[4] *Ibid.*, p. 977.

cism by fellow practitioners or experts in order to protect the interests of those who are supposed to be served. Patently, solo practice, in which a physician sets up an office and treats patients without visibility or any apparent accountability to anyone but himself, is not acting in accordance with these service ideologies. Similarly, suppression of internal criticism of fellow practitioners on the basis of a belief in the inviolability of judgments formed from individual experience, and on the basis of the argument that the critic was not present at the time, is not in keeping with these ideologies. To state that, under certain social conditions of low population density and rarity of physicians (a net shortage of physicians), solo practitioners are indispensible if any medical services are to be available is one thing; to idealize the solo practitioner as a preferred form of practitioner organization is another.

This idealization of the individual practitioner is well explained by monopolization theory; it represents a denunciation of organized forms of practice and evidently leads the attack on organized forms of competition. The ideal of individual competition is actually a call for a return to the social terms of a fraternal guild-type of monopolization, in which the complexities of suppressing internal competition are minimal. Even though it manifestly calls for individual competition, it ironically demands noncompetition between individualized practitioners. The image of individual competition is a businessman's ideology which has been starkly borrowed for its external political value of drawing on popular anticorporation sentiments.

Such idealization of the individual practitioner represents an uneasiness on the part of the organized profession with regard to the efficacy of ethics as constraints on economic conduct. Implicit in a refusal to engage in organized practice forms is the belief that organized practitioners will fail to honor norms calling for noncompetition. In recent years, the ideal of the individual practitioner has declined somewhat, as witnessed by the growth of group practices, and this decline can be explained in terms of the profession's interest pursuits. Simply, it becomes superfluous when price undercutting becomes unlikely due to either professional solidarity or an overwhelming net shortage of physicians. A blanket refusal to engage in organized practice can be modified into a demand for practitioner control, as long as there is some reason to believe that practitioners will maintain a noncompetitive position. Within the context of this belief, certain types of organized practice became acceptable to organized medicine. Thus, the secular trend of the American organized profession has been to shift from shutting down competitive opportunities by demanding direct physician-patient term setting and no third-party interference, to demanding third-party arrangements under professional control.

The recent upsurge in popular demand for medical services in the face of a relatively restrictive medical supply economy only serves to reduce the organized profession's fear of competition from organized practice by making the price of care expensive everywhere. A net shortage of physicians can drive physicians' incomes sufficiently high to make fee fixing unnecessary.

The demand for purely fee-for-service compensation is also related to the threat of competition from organized practitioners. While salaries can maintain incomes equal to those under fee-for-service, the profession's experience with contract practice suggests the impoverishing effects they can have. There are other considerations as well. The idealization of the individual practitioner, intimately associated with the guild concept of monopolization, logically calls for a fee-for-service system, for it is the only major type of monetary remunerative method which does not require some form of administration for payment. Salaries and capitation fees require some type of central treasury. Obviously, these controllers are less vulnerable than the patient and so are in a less disadvantageous position with respect to the physician. The other major consideration is that fee-for-service payment maintains the price leadership of the medical societies, whether in the form of fee schedules or usual and customary payment. Organized practice might alter this situation considerably by permitting employing organizations to set the terms of employment.

In light of these relationships, it is not surprising to find
that the AMA has frequently opposed forms of organized
practice. In 1932, for instance, the AMA officially opposed
group practice despite the recommendation of the majority
report of its own Committee on the Cost of Medical Care
that medical practice should be reorganized into group practices financed by public insurance, taxation, or both methods.
Instead, it adopted the minority report's recommendation
that private insurance plans be developed for medical care.[5]
Beginning in the 1930's, the AMA also opposed "contract
practice," wherever physicians were salaried to provide unlimited services: specialty clinics such as the Mayo and Lahey
Clinics; a medical cooperative in Oklahoma under Dr. Mi-
chael Shadid; the Ross-Loos Clinic in Los Angeles; the Group
Health Association in Washington, D.C. (which led to the
successful prosecution of the AMA for conspiracy to engage
in restraint of trade); and the Health Insurance Plan of
Greater New York in 1954.[6] In none of these instances was
either the quality of care or the level of remuneration an
issue.

The AMA has also consistently opposed any governmental
participation in the organization of physicians. In 1920, it
officially opposed any subsidies for health centers, group
medicine, and diagnostic clinics by state or national governments. After World War One, it opposed "compulsory"
insurance plans financed by the government, continued its
opposition throughout the Truman administration, and was
unsuccessful only in 1965 against Medicare and Medicaid,
the nationally-financed insurance and subsidy programs for
the elderly and the welfare eligible.

The reform movement within the AMA

Since the AMA's political defeat on Medicare/Medicaid,
it has apparently faced the problem of recouping losses in
terms of public reputation incurred during the fight against
the legislation. The fight seems to have made the AMA's

[5] Odin W. Anderson, *The Uneasy Equilibrium* (New Haven: College & University
Press, 1968), pp. 95-99.
[6] *Ibid.*, pp. 157-161.

monopolistic strategy more publicly conspicuous, for certain reformers in the AMA have raised the question of how the AMA can become less monopolistic in the near future. Yet the apparent antimonopolistic position may only be a call for the AMA to act *less recognizably* monopolistic. The medical profession may come to appear less monopolistic but in fact become more so.

This reform faction within the AMA has sought to win AMA power to implement new policies. Assembled from the liberal state societies among certain of the most populous states, most notably New York and California, it has tried to use current public pressure to advance both its own power interests and its view of the public's interest in improved medical care. Its strongest appeal within the profession has been the argument that if the profession does not bring about publicly desired reforms, nonprofessionals will.

In 1965, the reform faction called for the creation of an AMA Committee on Planning and Development (COPD), which was set up in 1968. In July 1970, the COPD issued "The Himler Report," which was reviewed by AMA reference committees at the AMA national convention in Chicago. The political goals of this document were to issue a reform platform for the medical profession and to embarrass the incumbent leadership of the AMA. At the same time, it faced the difficult problem of not repudiating the AMA's traditional legitimacy by attacking past policies and tactics. Since the long-range goals of the reform faction have incorporated the AMA's historical trend toward a concentration of power, its recommendations carefully compromise an attack on policy with a defense of present structure.

The AMA's leadership accepted "The Himler Report" with gestures of openness, but subsequently sent individual recommendations separately to reference committees for review. In this way, the fate of the report became relatively invisible, giving some reformers the initial misinformed impression that the report had been accepted and recommended for approval to the House of Delegates of the AMA.[7] As it happened,

[7] Interview with Peter Libby, medical student and delegate to the 1970 AMA national convention in Chicago, Illinois, August 1970.

only two of twenty were approved, and these were the least controversial items. Four others were referred for further committee examination, and ten were rewritten. Three resolutions were divided into parts, so that two additional parts were approved, two were referred, and two rewritten. The fate of the recommendations referred to other committees was uncertain, since the content of these recommendations could be tabled indefinitely for further study.

The rewritten recommendations tended to follow the recommendations of the COPD Minority Report submitted by John H. Budd, M.D., who was subsequently elected as a Trustee. Inasmuch as this position is one of the most powerful within the inner circle of the AMA, one may assume that his recommendations during the period of his candidacy reflected the interests and opinions of the most powerful members of the AMA. The recommendations of the reference committees also probably reflected the opinion of the AMA's leadership, and if so, the function of referral to further committees becomes more apparent. By referring the documents, the reference committee could admit uncertainty about the political implications of the recommendations and so pass them upward in the hierarchy of policy making. Some were sent to the Council on Medical Service, but part of one very controversial item was sent to the Board of Trustees "for transmittal to appropriate councils and committees."[8] Though what the Board of Trustees in fact did with this recommendation is secret, it may well have been submitted to the core leadership for political review.

In addition to fragmenting the reformers, the AMA tried to present itself as though it had accepted recommendations from "The Himler Report," presumably to show its openmindedness and receptivity to diverse opinion within the medical profession. A number of substitutions for the original recommendations were made, the basis for many of them as laid out in Budd's Minority Report: "I also find a good deal of the basic tone unacceptable to me, and, I expect,

[8] "Report of the Council on Planning and Development (The Himler Report)," (American Medical Association, mimeographed copy, July 1970), reference committee D, p. 3, line 20.

to the House of Delegates, notably the air of apology and self-denunciation which pervades some of the Report."[9] Many recommendations were changed to eliminate criticism of past policies or actions of the AMA. Others were reworded as reaffirmations of existing AMA policies. To the superficial observer, many of the substitutions were little more than face-saving techniques of the AMA; many of them, however, constituted substantially different positions on the issues. At issue, in fact, was the very role and structure of the medical profession in American society in the future.

"The Himler Report," then, is an organizational platform which has so far not been adopted by the AMA. Yet it is interesting as an innovative and plausible concept of the direction which the AMA and the medical profession in the United States might go and as a suggestion as to what a new strategy of monopolization might be. As in the New York Medical Society versus AMA dispute of the late 1880's, the factions representing "The Himler Report" are again debating which line of monopolistic development the organized medical profession should follow.

An overview of the reform program

The reformers have found a way to provide what they believe is better medical care and at the same time a way to enrich and strengthen the profession. After Medicare was passed, many physicians, despite bitter initial opposition, discovered that the government had made available a large, guaranteed body of funds for medical services. Fears of governmental interference and loss of perogatives have not been realized to any significant extent. These recent experiences have been the basis for the reform movement: to draw on tax revenue guarantees of payment for services. In effect, this would create a new source of income for the profession and do away with the insecurity, inconvenience, and office expense of collecting bills from individual patients. It also helps cope with the profession's public image as a monopoly.

With a new source of income, doctors might provide more

[9] *Ibid.*, Minority Report, p. 1, lines 12-14.

care for more people and not appear to discriminate as much on the basis of the ability to afford care. Also, many patients would no longer need to pay the doctor directly; whatever hostility this business relationship might generate could be displaced onto the agency of payment, presumably agencies for tax collection or the government. For years doctors have feared regulation by third-party institutions, but they have also found that public anger at high fees can be directed at insurance companies for incomplete coverage rather than at the profession for high fees. The gains of increasing income into the profession through tax-supported programs cannot be underestimated. For many years the proponents of so-called "socialized medicine" were concerned with mechanisms of payment for services when patients could not afford them. The British National Health Service of 1948 has demonstrated, however, that to think of medical services as a fixed body of costs is naive. Medical services have been found to be in infinite demand; even more important, they are infinitely innovative and complex. Essentially, there can be as many medical services as there are funds available. No patient can receive too much attention or too many tests "just to be sure" or too many sophisticated instruments for diagnosis and treatment. All of these expenditures are easily justified as improvements in patient care. Also, as the complexity of these tasks increases, the medical profession can claim that it is entitled to higher fees because of its increased responsibility and skill. By providing technically superior and more personally satisfying services, the doctor becomes a socially more significant person and can make claims on society for greater rewards.

The reformers also wish to extend control of medical activities to other health-related workers as well as the medical profession; they wish to make policy not only for themselves but for other professionals as well. Whether these proposed changes will improve the quality of medical care is, of course, unknown. Nevertheless, one can predict some of the more likely political and organizational changes which they will bring.

The shape of reform is expansive: to add a new source

of income to the existing medical market. It does not propose to eliminate private practice, because such a move would elicit great opposition from doctors and because private practice has proven to be profitable. On the other hand, the reformers must be able to deliver enough medical manpower to take on the responsibilities of new, tax-supported programs. If too many doctors remain in private practice, they cannot meet this obligation vis-à-vis the federal government. Therefore, the strategy of reform tends toward increased control of medical practitioners and policy making by the AMA. The traditional bias of the decentralized system of state medical societies is an obstacle to establishing reform programs, and overcoming this necessarily calls for some means of circumventing internal democratic processes. The challenge is to make the AMA more than a mere political arm of the interests of the state medical societies.

The goals of the reformers, then, are a new source for income, a government-profession coalition to ensure payment of services, subordination of other health professions to form a "health team" with the organized medical profession at the "head of the health pyramid," preservation of traditional professional rights of the medical profession, ideologies which convince the public that these changes will be in a less monopolistic direction, and tightening up of AMA controls over the medical profession. Finally, the plan entails the development of legitimate means for domination of the other health professions of the "health team." It is important to examine these goals in detail, for they constitute the components of a new type of monopolization strategy.

A new source for income

"The Himler Report" reflects the problems of meeting an expanding public demand for medical services which the market cannot sustain. Rising consumer expectations of what can be hoped for from modern medical knowledge has damaged the profession's public image, because services are apparently not delivered on account of existing patterns of payment and physician organization. Public pressure for professional change, interestingly enough, lays the foundation for building a more tightly organized and powerful profession and extending economic relationships beyond the present market.

The report prefaces its platform by linking public discontent with an appeal for restructuring the profession: ". . . if the total health establishment is to meet the requirements and expectations of the public, it becomes mandatory that the individual professionals and the institutions that render health services be more closely organized and at a higher level than is now the case."[10] At the same time the report calls for the creation of a general health policy for the AMA and asks how many of the new health demands it should take on. Admitting that no one yet has acquired authority for organizing health services, and that the "AMA has neither the facilities nor the personnel to undertake a regulatory and planning function on this scale," it argues that "both the interests of the public and those of the medical profession now require that the AMA and its constituent societies become actively involved in an endeavor to bring order and continuity to this presently chaotic field."[11] Hence, the interests of the AMA lie in the direction of controlling the organization of activity in the entire health market. The COPD therefore recommends: "That the AMA adopt an active role and take the initiative in developing *all* plans and programs for health care in *all* their ramifications and that it encourage and assist state and county medical societies to do the same at their respective levels."[12]

The COPD also recommends the relatively broad definition of health suggested by the World Health Organization: "Health is a state of complete physical, mental and social well-being and not merely the absence of disease or infirmity."[13] Furthermore, "that definition will establish the dimensions of the health care field in which the Association will function."[14] The COPD calls for the AMA to plan policy

[10] "COPD," AMA, *op. cit.*, p. 4.
[11] *Ibid.*, p. 6.
[12] *Ibid.*, p. 7.
[13] *Ibid.*, p. 6.
[14] *Ibid.*, p. 5.

in health matters, to create a system of health priorities, and to establish a "Health Bill of Rights" for consumers. Not only is this list of priorities wide ranging, covering everything from "continuous monitoring of health, growth, and development from birth to adult life" to "a healthful environment,"[15] but it would provide a mandate for the profession to claim additional resources from the government to close the gap between reality and ideals.

> Since the principle of comprehensive care has been generally accepted, it is important to determine precisely what services represent minimum acceptable and optimum levels. If the resources are available to supply all services representing optimum care simultaneously and immediately, there is no major problem. If, on the other hand, those resources are not at hand, it becomes necessary to evaluate all services in terms of their importance, urgency, and cost effectiveness, and to establish minimum standards and priorities on that basis.[16]

It would be, in effect, a means of ensuring the infinite expansion of the market for services in accordance with whatever policies the AMA might want to push. Whenever physicians could take on additional responsibilities and increase income for the profession, more elaborate and complex programs could be constructed. Whenever physicians are overloaded, the AMA can always fall back on the concept of priorities: the most important goals must first be achieved within the resources provided by the public. The AMA can thus be provided with a means of demanding whatever it wishes from the public in the name of better health services without being held responsible for deficiencies.

Because of this dissociation of accountability from policy making, and because of the close relationship between availability of tax money and the provision of health services, legislators and not the profession can become the target of public discontent over health services. The minority report objected to this reasoning: "Assuming responsibility for con-

---

[15] *Ibid.*, p. 35.
[16] *Ibid.*, p. 34.

ditions which appear well beyond the influence and control of the AMA is to invite more criticism of the medical profession when their impossibility of attainment becomes evident."[17] As the immediate providers of health care, physicians might well be the first targets of public hostility. As the minority report goes on to say, "The current vilification of physicians generally for those Medicare inequities, costs and abuses for which the medical profession has little or no responsibility is disheartening."[18] In any event, the medical profession might run the danger of currying public disfavor for falling short of the responsibility it has claimed for itself. The idea of priorities might be used ideologically to deflect hostility, but undoubtedly other ideologies would have to be created. Only to the extent that the medical profession could persuade the public that it is the public's defender would it be successful.

The expansionist aims of the reformers are also evident in their statement of primary purpose and responsibility:

> To endeavor, by all appropriate means, to make health services of high quality available to all individuals, in a dignified and acceptable manner, regardless of their social class, ethnic origin, ability to pay for services, or the source of the payment.[19]

According to Reference Committee A, "Witnesses questioned the practicality or advisability of committing the Association to a purpose which could exceed the capability of the profession and which entered areas outside professional control."[20] The Committee substituted the following:

> That the AMA reaffirm, as a statement of the primary purpose and responsibility of the Association and the medical profession, "the promotion of the art and science of medicine and the betterment of public health," and,

---

[17] "COPD," AMA, *op. cit.*, Minority Report, p. 2.
[18] *Ibid.*, p. 4.
[19] *Ibid.*, p. 3.
[20] "Actions Taken by the AMA House of Delegates at Its Recent Annual Convention," (American Medical Association, Mimeographed copy, 13 July 1970), pp. 9-10.

as part of this purpose, apply all possible effort to make medical services of high quality available to all individuals.[21]

Aside from the manifest fear of public disappointment, the substitution suggests other issues. Fundamentally, the AMA's leadership is committed to its present type of monopolization strategy, which rests on a notion of intensive care for single patients rather than extensive care for many patients. The leaders apparently see that adoption of social utilitarian standards would endanger the kind of intensive, concentrated care that can be delivered to individual patients in a private, one-to-one relationship. In this sense if expansion is to occur, it is always to be within the claim that "high quality" care is being provided to all treated patients. Presumably, if high quality care cannot be provided to a patient, no care should be. The AMA substitution clearly leaves open the conditions which would compromise the quality of care to patients, omitting mention of any of the probable organizational changes that would come about with the adoption of governmental subsidies, such as the source of payment and social origin of patients. The AMA's choice of words here—"reaffirm"—reveals the basic intent of the leadership to sustain the traditional professional structure.

Yet even in the very important recommendation number eight, the COPD never attacks private practice per se. It calls on the AMA to cease praising private practice as superior to all other forms of care, but not to eliminate private practice. Number eight recommends, in part:

(1) That the Association take no public position for or against private solo practice, private group practice, closed panel group practice, fee-for-service payment, or prepayment by capitation. . . .
(3) That the Association, in all public statements, emphasize the concept that differences in education, culture and income levels create problems that may neces-

[21] *Ibid.*

sitate different systems of delivering medical care for different population groups.[22]

Reference Committee A's substitution is striking. Five of the seven parts of recommendation eight are omitted, and their significance will be discussed below. The two that remain alter the meaning of the proposed recommendations and illuminate which hidden issues are really at stake:

(1) In seeking as its goal the highest quality and availability of patient care, the American Medical Association advocates factual investigation and objective experimentation in new methods of delivery of health care, while still maintaining faith and trust in the private practice of medicine and pride in its accomplishments. (2) That the Association, in appropriate public statements, emphasize the concept that differences in education, state laws, culture and income levels create problems that may necessitate different systems of delivering medical care for different population groups and different geographic areas.[23]

Though superficially similar, the first part of the substitution absolutely reverses the meaning of the COPD recommendation by praising private practice.

The issue which emerges is the role of private practice should government employment be explored. The reformers leave considerable room for private practice to continue, but they realize that a health empire cannot be built on a decentralized, uncoordinated basis. They do not wish to do away with private practice, for fear of engendering hostility from the majority of private practitioners and eliminating an independent economic center of power, potentially very useful for pressing claims against the government and consumer groups. In negotiating, since the profession will not use strikes for fear of damaging its reputation, it must have

[22] "COPD," AMA, *op. cit.* (n. 8, above), p. 20.
[23] *Ibid.*, reference committee A, p. 9, lines 14-26.

a means of providing care without placing itself in a disadvantageous bargaining position. Private practice provides a means for doing this because it lets practitioners threaten to withdraw from public employment, providing a morally tenable retreat through the private distribution of services.

The reformers realize how the idea of intensive care can be a useful second-line defense while it explores the interest-advantages of extensive-care models of health care delivery. The changes in the second part of the substitution include replacing "all" with "appropriate" and adding the criteria of state laws and differences in geographical areas. Both work against changes in the current professional structure. "Appropriate" provides a loophole for not emphasizing the universal service concept, and "state laws" calls for taking into account legislation in some states that restricts the kinds of health delivery systems that may be organized. In some states, for instance, there is no facilitating legislation for Blue Cross or Blue Shield plans. Other states make types of organization other than private practice very difficult to establish. "State laws" and "geographical areas" would seem to favor the still controversial discriminatory practices of some states against racial groups; abeyance to them would contribute toward preserving the differences in amount and quality of care available to "second-class citizens" in many American states. The inclusion of maintaining local authority also seemingly works against the creation of a uniform national policy. A national policy, of course, is the reformers' main means for controlling the development of new forms of employment. Indeed, the organized profession's appropriation, through the idea of health rights and priorities, of the right to define health problems may be the most important mechanism of the reform strategy. As health experts, they can claim that they are the legitimate authorities in deciding what should be done.

Building the health pyramid

Because the reformers oppose dissociating medical from health activities, they must create a network of interdepen-

dent health professionals and supporting agencies, headed
if not entirely at least in the main by the organized medical
profession. This network, the "health team," is complex and
commensurately expensive; though it may create a greater
number of more sophisticated techniques of care, it can
increase the amount of wealth coming into the hands of the
medical profession—if it can keep the number of physicians
relatively low and place them in top positions of control.
Toward these goals, the reformers have explored qualitative
as well as quantitative changes in health organization, as,
for instance, in recommendation number six:

(2) That the Association, in its future declarations and
activities directed toward the alleviation of shortages
in health services and personnel, underscore the fact that
these shortages are not due merely to an insufficient
number of health professionals across-the-board, and
emphasize that maldistribution of practitioners geo-
graphically, by profession, and by specialty is an equally
important factor in depriving communities of an adequate supply and spectrum of health services.[24]

The reformers therefore call, first, for the creation of a
body of personnel with medium-level skills to free doctors
from many routine tasks: physician's assistants, registered
nurses trained in well-baby care, army medical corpsmen,
and midwives. To justify domination of these paramedical
health professionals, however, the reformers then point out
the dangers in this system: possible "significant deterioration
of services" without physician supervision, increased malpractice suits against physicians for errors committed by
assistants, and increased depersonalization of care. The conclusion drawn on the basis of these "dangers" is revealing:

This expedient, if generally adopted, would be applied
to a great number of specialties and would result in the
creation of a number of sub-professions which would
be a nightmare to license, limit, audit and supervise.

[24] *Ibid.*, p. 15.

Understandably, but inevitably, the new assistant groups would seek to widen the permissible scope of their services and to increase their responsibility, authority, remuneration, and independence of action. This could seriously compromise physicians' responsibility for the care of their patients, and materially increase the cost of that care. The medical profession must not fall into the error of accepting the principle of creating corps of "doctors' assistants" except with stringent safeguards and provision for their close supervision.[25]

The Committee therefore recommends:
(1) That an appropriate Committee of the AMA immediately begin to formulate policy on doctors' assistants, particularly with regard to their responsibilities, limitations on their practice, and supervision of their services by qualified physicians.
(2) That the AMA reaffirm the principle that the basic responsibility for the care and welfare of patients lies with their physicians of record and that responsibility cannot and should not be delegated.[26]

In short, structural differentiation of health services is acceptable only as long as authority remains in the hands of the medical profession.

Dealing with health professionals and groups already long in existence poses a different problem of control. Although physicians' assistants can be controlled by creating them through a downward delegation of responsibility from the medical profession, these other groups can be controlled only by overcoming longstanding suspicion and relative autonomy. Currently, many hospitals already manage such problems as the admission of private patients, the use of patients for teaching purposes, and the distribution of government funds. The organized medical professions, to protect its interests, logically should go as far as possible to establish the principle that its interests should be taken into account

[25] *Ibid.*, p. 16.
[26] *Ibid.*, pp. 16-17.

by these relatively autonomous hospitals. The report seems to grasp this relationship:

> The medical associations have no direct authority over hospitals and, generally speaking, the attending physicians at each institution must work out their own formula for their relationships with each other and with their hospital. The hospital associations are similarly limited in their authority over member hospitals. Nevertheless, in some areas the medical societies and the corresponding hospital associations have been able to agree on some basic principles that apply to these staff situations and are gradually prevailing on hospital administrations to accept them. This is a slow and roundabout process but it seems to be the only way to regularize these complex relationships and restore peace and stability to hospital staff function.

> The Committee therefore recommends:
> (1) That the Association secure data from state and county medical societies on problems in physician-hospital relationships in their areas and the measures, if any, that are being taken to solve them.
> (2) That, on the basis of these data, the Association identify the basic principles that apply to staff-hospital relationships and encourage state and county medical societies to do the same.
> (3) That the Association and each state and county medical society request its counterpart in the hospital association structure to assist in developing guidelines and urge their member associations and hospitals to implement them.[27]

The reformers in the organized medical profession particularly wish to retain control over the emerging health pyramid with respect to the handling of governmental subsidies. When the act providing for Medicare-Medicaid (PL 89-97) was passed, the organized medical profession preferred to

[27] *Ibid.*, p. 30.

have payments handled through the Blue Plans (Blue Cross and Blue Shield) because, in the words of "The Himler Report," "the Blue Shield Plans were existing, functioning entities with a known capacity for program administration, ... their requirements, forms and procedures were familiar to the physicians who had supported their programs through the years," they would decrease transitional "confusion and delays," the National Association of Blue Shield Plans (NABSP) had already advocated the profession-approved concept of usual and customary prevailing rate (UCPR) fees, and "The final, and perhaps most significant factor in the adoption of this policy by the profession, was the belief that the Blue Plans were receptive to the thinking and wishes of physicians since after all the medical profession had majority representation on the boards of directors of most plans."[28] The AMA was disappointed to find, however, that the Blue Plans under Medicare were mostly administrative and advisory agencies and that final policy decisions were made by the Social Security Administration and the Department of Health, Education, and Welfare.

The influence that the medical societies hoped to exercise over the Title 18 and Title 19 *Medicare-Medicaid* programs, through their close association with the Blue Shield Plans, has therefore proved to be illusory.[29]

It has become clear that what medicine hoped to use as a buffer between itself and government has become an insulator. The Committee is of the opinion that such insulation is undesirable and that all medical societies should seek to establish and maintain open, direct channels of communication with the agencies that set policy for government health programs.[30]

A liaison committee between the AMA and the NABSP was founded after the 1967 NABSP meeting because "some

[28] *Ibid.*, pp. 30-31.
[29] *Ibid.*, p. 31.
[30] *Ibid.*, p. 32.

Blue Shield Plans have been showing a tendency to deal directly with the physicians in their area and to circumvent the medical societies that represent those physicians. . . . The Committee is of the opinion that, at this time, when the entire system of providing and paying for health services is under critical public appraisal, the relationships between the medical profession and the Blue Shield and Blue Cross Plans should be close, cordial, and cooperative."[31] What prompted the COPD to call for a tightening of professional controls over these health service administrative agencies is suggested in this commentary from the report:

> To summarize this topic, the Blue Shield Plans are changing in their fundamental nature in response to pressures from government, from consumers and from the Blue Cross Plans with which they are associated. Their dependence on the medical profession has diminished, and they are generally less responsive to the opinions and the guidance of the medical societies. The loosening of ties is further aggravated by the long tenure of most of the medical members of the boards of directors who, having outgrown their society ties, no longer reflect current medical policy and often fail to alert their medical societies to changes in Blue Shield operations and their significance. The stresses to which our health care system is currently being subjected call for new and imaginative approaches to the utilization and distribution of our total pool of resources in terms of manpower, facilities, and money, if voluntary systems are to survive. Blue Cross, Blue Shield, and the Association all have a vital interest in voluntarism in health care. That joint interest calls for them to close ranks and coordinate their efforts and their planning.[32]

The health pyramid, then, is to be a network of newly created assistant groups closely supervised by the organized medical profession, hospitals in which the interests of the

[31] *Ibid.*, p. 33.
[32] *Ibid.*

medical profession are protected by mutual agreement with
hospital associations, and payment administrative bodies
responsive to the organized medical profession because of
common interests.

Other groups not as closely related to the health professions may also be made part of the pyramid. The report
discusses the Partnership for Health Act (PL 89-749) in
relation to the problems of authority, advice, and consumer
participation. This law "provides federal matching funds for
the development and operation of Health Planning Commissions under which the state and regional agencies for comprehensive areawide health planning will function." Many
regions report having difficulties because of "bickering"
among constituent groups, the most important of these,
apparently, being the local authorities and the health professions. "The local government, in these instance, attempts
to gain control of the planning council and exercises its veto
power over other proposals for agencies with wide community
representation."[33]

The organized medical profession's greatest opponent, apparently, in its attempt to build a health pyramid under
its direction and control, is government at all levels. The
only way for it to oppose governmental control is to replace
it with both professional and consumer control. The AMA
reformers seem quite convinced that the government, particularly at the federal level, is in principle opposed to listening
to organized medicine. Only by developing sympathetic ears
elsewhere in consumer groups can the AMA overcome governmental control in the absence of majority professional
representation:

The ultimate fate of public, or consumer, participation
in health care planning, as embodied in the Partnership
for Health Amendments, is also difficult to foretell at
this early date. There is growing evidence, however, that
government health agencies will resist more than token
involvement of the public in planning, as they have
resisted that of organized medicine. It begins to appear

[33] *Ibid.*, pp. 36-37.

that the so-called Areawide Comprehensive Health
Planning agencies will be mere reshufflings of the same
groups and individuals who are now influential with
government, health and hospital administrative authorities. If the communities and the medical profession
permit this to happen, planning for health services may
be dominated or completely controlled by government
health agencies and officials. As a consequence, strong
pressure would be exerted for the expansion of prepaid
group practice while private solo and group practice,
based as they are on fee-for-service payments, would
become the targets for regulation and fee control. The
importance of properly balanced representation of all
competent and interested segments of the population
on comprehensive health planning bodies is quite clear,
since only such broadly based organizations will permit
the various health service delivery systems to prove their
worth in competition with one another.[34]

The reformers believe that the consumer groups can be
easily coopted by organized medicine. The law (PL 89-749)
states that there must be at least 51 percent consumer
representation in such administrative systems; if these
groups were persuaded to see things from the perspective
of the professional groups, governmental control could be
effectively avoided. "Many consumer and community groups
do not yet have individuals to represent them who are
experienced, well informed, and have the vision to look
beyond immediate factional interests. Such representation
takes time to develop and its lack will delay the achievement
of effective planning. Nevertheless, the intent of the law is
clear and these groups should be incorporated into the
planning commissions and encouraged and assisted in every
way."[35] Considering that the AMA reformers propose creating an extensive data-collection and analysis center for the
purpose of policy making, it would appear that they would
be able to "educate" the consumer groups with their own

[34] *Ibid.*, p. 40.
[35] *Ibid.*, p. 37.

evaluation of how different health delivery systems worked out "in competition."

Yet by conceding 51 percent representation to consumer groups, organized medicine would deny itself ultimate authority in the design of health systems. The reformers might be able to coopt consumer representatives, but if they do not, they might well lose control of the planning councils. Not surprisingly, then, the minority report opposed 51 percent consumer representation, even the unnecessary "gratuitous endorsement" in the concession by the majority report that "the intent of the law is clear."[36] Yet the disclaimer suggests that the COPD's support of consumer groups is more than cooptative *Realpolitik*. If the health pyramid is to draw on governmental sources of income, it must work within the legal framework imposed by the governmental agencies which fund programs. Since majority consumer representation is a condition imposed by the legislature, and since such representation would make organized medicine appear less monopolistic than would its own majority representation, establishing a strong tradition of persuasive influence and thereby domination over the consumer groups could achieve many ends desirable to the reformers.

Establishing professional authority

Even though on the issue of consumer representation the medical reformers have appeared to surrender one policy-making right for the sake of coopting the newly created planning councils, the AMA reformers do not plan to lose control of policy making. Even without official majority control, they can represent their interests by establishing nonnegotiable criteria to defend the profession's interests and by initiating aid in planning new services by other groups. The five sections of recommendation number eight which were omitted in the Reference Committee's substitution illustrate how the AMA could determine health policy as health experts without being conspicuously in control:

[36] *Ibid.*, Minority Report, p. 5.

(2) That an appropriate committee of the AMA be charged with the task of establishing the basic criteria which any proposed system of delivery of health services or mechanism for payment must satisfy to be acceptable. . .

(4) That the state and local medical societies be encouraged and assisted in devising and proposing practice expedients suited to their localities and their problems.

(5) That the Association, in conjunction with the state and county medical societies, establish a consultation and assistance service for physicians or groups of physicians who wish to develop organizations or programs for the rendering of health services.

(6) That the AMA endeavor to be informed of the pilot projects that are proposed by other sources and that it request the Department of HEW to discuss those projects with the Association before they are put into effect.

(7) That the Association seek to insure that the value judgments made by the Department of HEW on plans, programs, pilot projects and payment mechanism are firmly based on the criteria and standards the AMA has developed for that purpose.[37]

Implementation of these criteria, perhaps in the form of a detailed health policy or "Health Bill of Rights," is the means for extending domination to include health professionals who are not physicians, consumer groups, and even the Department of Health, Education, and Welfare. To this extent, the right to decide the structure of organized health care is linked with the right to define health problems.

The reformers, after all, reaffirm their belief in traditional professional policy-making rights. In licensing requirements, and the monitoring and policing of physicians' fees, the reformers retain policy making in the hands of the medical societies or institutional bodies amenable to medical society influence:

[37] "COPD," AMA, op. cit., p. 20.

The Committee is of the opinion that fee policing or, indeed, any other supervision of physicians is best kept in the medical societies. Peer judgments are much more likely to be just and equitable in these matters than are decisions made by outside agencies. At the same time, if the societies elect to make only the judgments and, by agreement, leave enforcement to government agencies, they may at some future time be excluded from both functions.

Again, the monitoring of fees does not fall within the province of the AMA but the Association should advise the state and county medical societies to assume that function and should assist them in securing the necessary powers.[38]

Attempts by those outside the profession to regulate the quality of medical practice, such as the demands for qualifications for specialists and postgraduate education for generalists made by the New York State Department of Health for Medicaid patients, are also opposed.

The mere existence of a double standard is undesirable and it seems logical and should be tightened. Once the determination has been made that this is the case, the drafting of new standards would best be accomplished by the cooperative efforts of the Board of Regents, the State Department of Health, and the State Medical Association.[39]

Monitoring and policing fees by the organized profession are consistent with both professional ideologies of self-regulation and the profession's traditional monopolistic right to set the value of services. The reformers prefer to retain the UCPR concept to prevent governmental tax-supported programs from undercutting private practitioners. Though patients may prefer a tax-supported program, physicians would not want their income reduced by participation in the pro-

[38] *Ibid.*, p. 23.
[39] *Ibid.*, p. 26.

gram. Yet charges that some physicians were abusing the program by overcharging for services or performing unwarranted services might discourage the government from paying for any services. So, uniform fees attain a new monopolistic significance: keeping open the new income source.

Indeed, such regulatory functions are quite compatible with progressive monopolization. If all physicians adhere to a homogeneous, rising UCPR fee schedule, then the profession can slowly increase its total income, though some members may have to forego short-term gains. The reformers' opposition to an educational double standard for physicians in private or tax-supported practices is also monopolistic. Since private practice is important for providing an independent center of power from which to negotiate with the government and to set base levels for fees, it should appear at least as attractive to patients as tax-supported programs. If government programs are known to require higher qualifications than private practice, private practice might become publicly identified with inferior care. A competitive advantage for governmentally-financed services is not in the monopolistic interests of the profession, of course, and though private practice would not necessarily mean inferior care, the public might believe that government programs guarantee a generally high level of care. In any event, the organized profession is not prepared to concede its authority over the determination of proper levels of qualification for medical practice in any setting.

The ultimate fate of private practice in the plans of the reformers is not discussed. They would like to maneuver the government into a position of paying for medical services on the organized profession's terms. To do this, the government and other interested parties have to recognize the organized profession's asserted rights to dictate fees, conditions of practice, educational requirements, and the like. To create such authority in the face of governmental opposition might require the strategic use of alternative private practice; once established, however, the authority could conceivably persist without the power base of private practice. The possibility that organized medicine might not be able to institutionalize such far-sweeping, monopolistic authority always remains, and the report is not clear about how such rights would be established.

The AMA leadership's experience with the government with respect to compulsory insurance plans led to the ideology that any participation of government in medical care would "inevitably" lead to socialized medicine.[40] Despite difficulties with the Department of Health, Education, and Welfare, the reformers believe that they can escape governmental domination by providing comprehensive medical care with the help of governmental subsidies. Implicitly, they do not accept the shibboleth that "he who pays the piper calls the tune." This difference is illustrated in the report in an exchange between the leadership (as represented in the minority report) and the reformers.

Reformers: "Physicians have always had an almost atavistic distrust and fear of government intrusion into any aspect of medical practice."[41]

AMA leadership: "The distrust and fear of government intrusion into medical practice, described as 'atavistic,' is indeed well founded and as justifiable as most primitive instincts."[42]

The hope of the reformers to institutionalize professional control over government subsidies is expressed in their position statement on the value of negotiation with the government:

It would certainly be useless, as well as contrary to the medical profession's traditions, for physicians or their representatives to adopt the trade union "bargaining" approach.

This does not mean, however, that negotiation is useless as a means of promoting or securing suitable conditions and reimbursement for physicians. It merely means that we must find an alternative to force or pressure to

[40] James G. Burrow, *AMA: Voice of American Medicine* (Baltimore: Johns Hopkins Press, 1963), p. 219.
[41] "COPD," AMA, *op. cit.* (n. 8, above), p. 31.
[42] *Ibid.*, Minority Report, p. 4.

reinforce our claims. The only logical alternative is to establish a climate in which medical associations and government agencies may agree to negotiate with mutual respect and a recognition of the community of their goals. Government has a powerful incentive to establish a smooth and cooperative relationship with the medical profession since physicians are required to implement all health programs and control the utilization of facilities and non-medical health personnel.[43]

What they envision, then, is a government-profession health coalition that would enlarge as well as maintain professional monopolistic privileges and provide government with the means of building the medical component of the new welfare state. The organized medical profession's opposition to welfare statism, then, could conceivably dissolve under conditions which did not damage professional interests.

Governmental subsidies, however, are limited by budgetary considerations. The medical profession would have to deal with organized collectivities instead of atomized individual consumers over subsidies. For the medical profession to retain the monopolistic authority to set the value of medical services, it should have a mechanism to take into consideration the budgetary limitations of governmental resources. The COPD tries to explain what function negotiation would play:

> Physicians sometimes have difficulty in understanding why, if the usual, customary, prevailing and reasonable concept is preserved, there should be a need for negotiation. Nevertheless, the fact that they shy away from the term "prevailing" and prefer to omit it from their writings and discussion indicates that there is either a conscious or instinctive recognition that the prevailing fee is actually an unpublished maximum fee schedule which can be set at any percentage of customary fees. It therefore follows that at some time negotiations to set the percentile of prevailing fees will become neces-

[43] *Ibid.*, p. 43.

sary. The parting remarks of the outgoing Secretary of
Health, Education, and Welfare substantiate this belief.
If existing medical societies fail to prepare themselves
for negotiation, other groups will inevitably take over
that function and thereby undermine the societies'
membership and influence.[44]

Negotiation serves a variety of functions, depending on the
political development of profession-government relationships. In its earliest phase, it provides an alternative method
to the doctors' strike for the acquisition of governmental
concessions with respect to the conditions of practice and
regulation as well as the payment of fees. At the same time,
it begins to establish the principle that the medical profession's interests should be taken into account in the creation
of new health care delivery systems. The organized profession
can then develop a distinction between negotiable and nonnegotiable with the understanding that some things are
supposedly so vital to the interests of the profession that
alternatives would not be acceptable. Finally, negotiation
provides an ongoing, institutionalized means for pressuring
the government for more budgetary allocations for medical
and health care programs.

The very word "negotiation" also plays an important
public-relations role. By claiming the right to have its interests taken into account in accord with "principles, ground
rules, and procedures," organized medicine opens the door
for expanding its sphere of de facto domination. Entering
negotiations provides the power basis for later establishing
professional control in other areas. By first establishing the
criteria that its claims are necessary for acceptability of a
program, the profession can shape the structure and operation of systems it could not otherwise regulate or adminis-
trate in any practical manner. Acceptance by government
agencies of the legitimacy of such criteria would extend the
profession's domination well into the public realm; yet the
arrangement would appear nonmonopolistic, since policies
would appear to be made by governmental agencies. This

[44] *Ibid.*, p. 44.

public presentation of independent governmental policy
making would provide the organized medical profession with
monopolistic control at a top level and a nonmonopolistic
image on a popular level. To the public, the profession would
present itself as a servant; to the government, it would
present itself as the health expert.

Building successful public relations

The American medical profession has never been as successful as it might wish in garnering public support. Kappa
Lambda, the first American medical society, had to meet
as a secret society to avoid criticism as a conspiracy. In 1811,
Baltimore magistrates would not convict unlicensed practitioners, and the public reportedly preferred irregular practitioners blacklisted by the examination boards.[45] Much of the
ideology generated by the American organized profession can
be related, I believe, to its attempts to distract public attention from its monopolistic features and to interpret its actions
as purely in the public's interest. While many in the AMA
apparently believe that the American public's distrust of the
medical profession is based on the AMA's politically-oriented
behavior during its opposition to the passage of Medicare
legislation, the AMA leadership does not believe that this
suspicion is justified; it believes that its opposition to Medicare was based on considerations of the public interest.
Whatever its actual motives were, the AMA currently faces
the central problem of how to deal with the manifestly
monopolistic appearance of its half-century-long opposition
to governmental subsidy of the expansion of health care,
and the public's interpretation of at least some of that
opposition as not being in the public interest.

The AMA has apparently come to accept Medicare as a
fact of life, has changed its official policy to permit at least
partial federal support of medical schools, and for some time
has supported federal funding for construction of health care

[45] Joseph F. Kett, *The Formation of the American Medical Profession: The Role
of Institutions, 1780-1860* (New Haven and London: Yale University Press, 1968),
p. 22.

facilities. In "The Himler Report," the reformers propose
to go even further to alter the public's image of professional
monopolistic behavior by entering into a coalition with the
government and ending the policy of opposition which pur-
portedly diminishes public support. Public support would of
course legitimize the profession's political gains and also
provide the profession with a tactical weapon in its negotiations with the government.

The report is remarkably frank about the intended use
of public relations. In a section entitled "Legislation: essential conditions for successful public relations and legislative
programs," it sets forth both method and rationale. Since
the "most important single requirement" is that the AMA
be "respected for its motivations and purposes," therefore
the AMA should adopt a general policy statement which
appears "demonstrably in the public interest." The statement early in the report, which calls for the distribution
of high quality health services to all individuals regardless
of ability to pay, source of payment, social status, or ethnic
origin, guided and assisted by the AMA, might serve such
a purpose. Subsequent specific policies should be innovative
and directed toward problem solving and correcting health
care deficiencies *that have been identified by the Association
itself.*" They should be "objective analyses of factual information" and not "subjective and emotional responses to
proposals made by officials or legislators," and should be
consistent with other policies and the general policy of the
AMA. To ensure favorable reception by legislators, however,
since "it is important to the AMA's public stature that it
be associated with as few failures as possible, each of its
statements, policies, and actions in the field of health service
legislation should be judged" according to four criteria:

(1) Is it in the public interest or interpretable as such?

(2) Is it politically advantageous, or at least innocuous
for the legislators to adopt?

(3) Will it have public support or, if controversial, is
it likely to have the support of a majority of politically
influential groups?

(4) Is it consistent with the previous policies and pro-

nouncements of the Association on the same or similar issues?[46]

Medicare, it goes on to say, is instructive in light of these criteria.

> The Association's opposition was more emotional than objective and was at least partially predicated on an underestimation of the problems faced by the elderly in the financing of health care. In spite of its honest motivation, the Association's position was easily distorted to give the impression that physicians were opposed to the provision of needed aid to the elderly for selfish reasons, obviously not in the public interest. In addition, the AMA's policy did not have the support of a majority of the populace and would therefore have been a liability for any legislator to espouse. About the only criterion it did meet was that of consistency with earlier positions on the same subject.[47]

In another passage from the report, the reformers more clearly outline the changes in ideology made necessary by public beliefs. They call for the AMA to end its single-minded support of private practice, especially the use of terms such as "private practice," "fee-for-service payment" and "free choice."

> The Committee is keenly aware of the virtues of many of our present methods of practice but their importance has not yet been proven to the public. Arguments directed toward establishing what has become almost a medical mystique fall on deaf ears in an era when a substantial number of our population depend on government assistance to buy health services and must, with the benefits provided, compete with other segments of society for services that are costly and in short supply. Until and unless the Association addresses itself publicly,

---

[46] "COPD," AMA, *op. cit.* (n. 8, above), p. 45.
[47] *Ibid.*, p. 46.

actively, and objectively to the resolution of the very concrete problems that exist in health care, its attempts to justify present delivery systems and payment mechanisms will be incomprehensible both to the public and government and will be interpreted as self-seeking on the part of the profession. The Association can and should strive to preserve those features of medical practice that it considers important, but the justification for so doing must be based on proofs of value that are meaningful to the lay public.[48]

In short, the current ideologies as well as much of the structure of the medical profession are not compatible with welfare-state politics.

Despite expansion and development of its interests, a reformed medical profession would still have to dissociate itself from certain traditional policies because of possible public opposition to self-interested policies. This position is argued in a recommendation in "The Himler Report" for the formation of a "National Academy of the Health Professions for Research and Policy." This proposed academy would be composed of representatives of national associations of health professions, paramedical professions, and national public health agencies. It would collect, analyze, and store data and generate policy recommendations that would carry the weight of the uniform consensus of all these health professions. The academy would serve three functions: (1) data and policies would not "bear the stigmata of professional prejudice and self-seeking," since they would represent the opinion of more than one organization; (2) broad participation in policy making would enhance interprofessional cooperation in the health pyramid; (3) legal entanglements of "interlocking directorates" would be avoided by divorcing "the academy completely from the politics of its parent societies. This is an essential condition without which the academy could not command the prestige and public confidence it must have to serve the purposes for which it is founded."[49]

[48] *Ibid.*, pp. 50-51.
[49] *Ibid.*, p. 57.

The report suggests, however, that the participation of other health professions in the academy would probably be token. "These groups would be unlikely to accept or take affirmative action on policies they had no part in developing. The AMA has recognized the advantages of coordinating its efforts with those of other professional associations but has not been able to bring those associations under the umbrella of its leadership."[50] The AMA would not relinquish control over policy making, for "policy formed by the academy, based on valid data, and developed in a continuous and logical manner, should almost invariably be acceptable to the House of Delegates and the Board of Trustees."[51] To this end, there would be "an additional weight or factor to the various organizations in determining their representation on the board of directors."[52]

The reformers believe that dissociation from health policies would free the AMA from "the stigma of trade unionism" and make recommendations more acceptable to the public.[53] The belief that a coalition of health profession associations could be more influential with public and government agencies reflects an awareness that the organized medical profession would lack the authority to dictate the structure and operation of health care delivery institutions. Such devices as the proposed health academy provide a tool for maintaining control over health policies in the absence of such authority. The reformers' proposed use of negotiation, criteria, and liaison committees also represents an attempt to dissociate exercised domination from authority, that is, to institute de facto domination. The only right claimed from the government and the public is that professional interests be taken into account in health planning. The structural framework constructed by the reformers would have the potential for ensuring that the profession would protect its own interests and exercise considerable control in determining the fate of health organization in the United States.

The right to set major policies is only one of a variety

[50] *Ibid.*, p. 54.
[51] *Ibid.*, p. 59.
[52] *Ibid.*, p. 56.
[53] *Ibid.*, p. 59.

of ways of furthering organized medicine's monopolistic interests. Ironically, maintaining a nonmonopolistic public image can further monopolistic control at the expense of monopolistic authority. Also, selectively entering into negotiations with the government to determine the conditions for subsidies may be nonmonopolistic in the sense that group success is increased only by wooing governmental favor; but the monopolistic advantages of accruing additional resources for the profession and creating new spheres of professional control make it a small price to pay.

Conceivably, the AMA could develop a strategy based on authority by virtue of expertise in health planning. In place of resting professional authority on its unique health care service skills, it might emphasize its planning ability as "head" of the health pyramid. The organized medical profession could draft a health plan and a budget that the government would be compelled to acknowledge as a "necessary" part of a welfare commitment, thereby maximizing income from the national government. Should welfare goals assume increasing importance as national goals, the profession could be in a favorable position. Similarly, establishing the value of the planning expertise of the organized medical profession could result in the acceptance of its authority by the other health professions. A differentiation of function between the medical profession as health planners and other health professions as implementers of those plans may well be in the future. Such developments would of course legitimize and institutionalize the new monopolization strategy.

Tightening up the medical profession

The reconstitution of the social role of the medical profession would also lead to changes within the profession. If organized medicine is to be the head of the health pyramid, it must generate policies and provide manpower for proposed programs. "The Himler Report" calls for a number of changes to make a detailed health policy possible. Its resolution to "adopt an active role and take the initiative in developing *all* plans and programs for health care in *all* their ramifications" is clearly a move in this direction.[54] Recommendation five calls on the AMA to "secure data from all the state medical societies on the adequacy of health services and the manner in which they are being provided in their rural and underprivileged areas, and the practice mechanisms, if any, that are being considered or developed to correct existing deficiencies. Based on this information, the same committee should devise delivery systems consonant with the Association's principles and incentives for physicians to settle in medically deprived localities."[55]

Similarly, the AMA should collect data and formulate policy on "manpower shortages,"[56] "medical fees,"[57] "physician-hospital relationships,"[58] and "the services that comprise comprehensive care"[59] as part of a "Health Bill of Rights." These policies tie together the "health team" with the medical profession at the top and exert pressure on the government to provide additional funding for health programs; they also present individual physicians with new types of demands from the organized profession. Once a policy is made and supported by the organized profession, it would be embarrassing not to fulfill the policy. The pressure to carry out policy then becomes a mandate for the organized profession to develop new mechanisms of internal control of its membership.

One such mechanism might be the use of "office audits" of quality of care. These already exist to varying degrees in certain hospitals; the use of computers could extend them into offices. Possession of "objective" evidence of the performance of individual physicians could be a powerful weapon for mobilizing cooperation through compliance. Fee monitoring and setting fee limits by the medical societies might also be methods for extending additional control over physicians.[60]

[54] *Ibid.*, p. 7.
[55] *Ibid.*, p. 14.
[56] *Ibid.*, p. 15.
[57] *Ibid.*, p. 22.
[58] *Ibid.*, p. 30.
[59] *Ibid.*, p. 36.
[60] *Ibid.*, p. 23.

In any event, one major goal of "The Himler Report" is the centralization of control in the hands of the AMA, thereby removing control from the state medical societies. To form a detailed health policy, the AMA must obtain for technical purposes comprehensive, standardized information on the behavior of physicians nation-wide. The present structure of the AMA is unconducive to this standard-ization, because each medical society collects data unsystem-atically. Even though the report calls for the preservation of the "basic elements of the Association's present struc-ture,"[61] it aims at greater centralization of control:

> . . . properly organized, the societies would form a nationwide network devoted to data accumulation and analysis. The Association's function should be to pro-mote the formation of these resources and to establish uniform standards as to the manner in which data are accumulated, reported, and forwarded. Even those county and state societies that are most jealous of their prerogative and autonomy will recognize the advantages offered by this course of action and will not consider it an invasion of their rights.

> An obvious corollary to this thesis is that the AMA must become more aggressive in its leadership and work ac-tively to create and coordinate the facilities and capabil-ities of these units of organized medicine so that they may serve a group function while retaining their individ-ual identities and purposes. In essence, the AMA must become a much tighter and more effective federation than it has been hitherto and the stimulus for such reorganization must be applied from above downward.[62]

Centralization would provide the AMA with the capacity for expansion and alteration of existing health functions to take advantage of new medical demands. It would also provide a more secure means for the reformers to assume

[61] *Ibid.*, p. 50.
[62] *Ibid.*, p. 52.

and hold control within the AMA. One reason for the stability of the AMA oligarchy during the twentieth century in the face of internal formal democracy has probably been the general consensus of values and interests among the Board of Trustees and the House of Delegates. One would anticipate considerable opposition to the reformers from the House of Delegates, who represent the interests of the state medical societies, should the reformers attempt to take power. The reformers would face the problem of establishing internal authoritative control in the national organization for the carrying out of a reform program; the majority of conservative state medical societies probably would be recalcitrant to "suggestions" from the national. Thus, the reformers require the creation of a national program that would legitimize subordination of the local societies. In essence, the internal structure of organized medicine would probably be transformed from a confederation into a federation by such an internal appropriation of domination by the reformers.

The Himler Report as a monopolization strategy

The most critical theoretical problem posed by the report is the sense in which it may be construed as monopolistic. It is unlike the model of monopolization which was presented earlier in that it is prepared to enlarge the supply of physicians, let physicians combine into organized practices, permit nonphysicians to share in the performance of medical services and to enter into economic agreements with organized consumer groups. It does not strictly restrict membership in the profession (in the sense of decreasing numbers), forbid the formation of potentially competitive interest groups within the profession, eliminate external competitors, or atomize consumers. In what respects, then, is the reform platform monopolistic?

The report is an interesting document because it proposes to push the group's collective interests through new organizational means. Instead of trying to maximize total group income through improving the group's competitive position in the market (by regulating supply), the report proposes to draw on governmental funds to raise more income than apparently is possible through market mechanisms (by expanding demand). In this sense—that it increases the group's potential for gain—it is theoretically more favorable to group success than the traditional AMA strategy.

The report is also a strategy of domination in that it relies heavily on group cooperation and organization. Despite permitting organized practices, the report does not suggest that physicians compete with one another. Therefore, it does not totally abandon older strategies: it does not encourage internal or external competition; it does not propose to eliminate licensure; and it recruits allied health professionals to perform certain traditional medical services only so that physicians can perform new functions, freeing themselves from the limitations imposed by their traditional monopolization strategy. Physicians will not compete with physicians' assistants and nurses; they will subordinate these auxiliary workers to the interests of physicians. Because the AMA would act as the central negotiating agent for the profession, according to the report, it would actually require more control of physicians to let the AMA enter into contracts with the government. In this sense, the amount of cooperation—even in the form of compliance—that the AMA would require would be greater than under the present decentralized, fraternalistic model of the profession.

An increase in physicians constitutes restriction of membership only in a narrowly absolute sense. Increasing income through governmental subsidies may raise not only the profession's total income but also the per capita income of physicians because of increased numbers of patients and demand for services which can be compensated. Thus, the "expanded" profession may be relatively restricted under new conditions for delivering services. Yet it is because the expansion of professional membership would extend domination over activities from which outsiders would be excluded that one can interpret this strategy as monopolistic. It is a plan to monopolize certain new activities over which the organized profession currently exerts no control.

Another means by which the report is monopolistic is its presentation as nonmonopolistic. By dissociating the AMA from traditionally recognizable monopolization tactics, the report superficially appears to be less monopolistic. The tactics it substitutes, however, are consistent with a new type of monopolization strategy, which the public does not consider monopolistic. Not only is this important for reducing popular opposition to the profession, but it helps prevent state intervention into the profession's control of the practice of medicine, at the same time ensuring continuing positive state privileges. As a method of restrictive domination (as an appropriation of certain supplies), therefore, the report is technically interpretable as monopolistic, even though the restriction of numbers of suppliers of services (closure) is not a prominent feature of the new strategy.

Reasons for shifting monopolization strategies

Why a new monopolization strategy in the context of contemporary American politics would "make sense" from the point of view of both the organized medical profession and those who control other institutions in America deserves some consideration. One can begin from the report's manifest explanation for a new strategy: if the organized medical profession should fail to bring about certain changes in medical care delivery, the government will do it. This "inevitability," however, is contingent on a great number of conditions, and so one should consider a number of other aspects of the program.

As suggested repeatedly in this chapter, the report is a program which does not undermine the collective interests of the medical profession in America but which may in fact promote them, by drawing on new sources of income and by further centralizing control of practitioner affairs in the hands of the AMA. A program which more effectively pushes the profession's collective interests would seem to be in itself an important explanation for shifting strategies. Yet merely being in the profession's interest is too general an explanation; it does not begin to explain why there has been a shift in strategy. For that, one logically requires a change to

explain a change. Apparently, the new strategy is an out-
growth of the profession's success with its old monopolization
strategy. The conventional market for medical services has
in some senses been exhausted by the organized profession's
tactics—the maximization of income by uniform fees and
restrictive policies, and the other monopolistic devices mentioned previously. To advance the profession's gain, organized medicine requires an expanded source of income which
can mobilize more income than can the market, which is
limited by considerations of individual demand and marginal
utility for services. Unlike the British divergence from the
RCP-type monopolization strategy because of failure to
dominate the market for medical services, the new American
strategy is a response to the limitations of relatively effective
monopolization.

There are contextual reasons as well. Winning more favorable public opinion is always in the profession's interest, but
a consideration of this type still does not answer what interest
controlling groups in America would have in a new type of
professional organization for medical services. One may be
satisfied with the general explanation of better medical care
for the American public, but that is still not dealing with
the issue of the interests of particular social groups in a
different structure for medical services. "The Himler Report"
has not yet been viewed from the perspective of the interest
constellation of the profession.

The central question is why ruling groups in America might
be interested in extending medical services to previously
"disenfranchised" social groups. I have offered one explanation for why the medical profession has been allowed to
persist as a monopolistic interest group: the additional
rewards for class success which it could provide for upper
classes. Now, even though one need not entirely abandon
this explanation, it cannot be accepted as adequate. In this
chapter, I have mentioned on several occasions the welfare-
statist aspects of the report's programs, ranging from the
need for governmental subsidies to a profession-government
coalition. Such a coalition might do more than merely further
legitimize the power of the government through welfare

activities or be a tool of the political parties for winning electoral votes (though certain prominent political figures have attempted to use the extension of coverage for medical services to win popular support). Welfare services might be used as a means for reducing popular discontent about class inequities or as a means for obviating popular political organization around obvious interest issues, [63] or they might be used as a means for controlling the lower classes by rewarding compliant conduct with adequate medical care.[64]

In fact, I find, the political interest of ruling groups in the extension of medical services is not at all clear; various degrees of Machiavellian speculation notwithstanding, my impression is that the extension of services will not reduce popular discontent beyond that directed at health issues, or necessarily prevent political organization of the masses, for medical care is a specific, not a general, political issue. Nor is a medical program, based on services for all regardless of social qualification (if it does what it says), a compatible program with a reward system for politically desired behavior from the lower classes, One of the political difficulties with "The Himler Report," indeed, is that within the American context, extending medical services may not be politically rational from the point of view of elite groups, except in those cases where specific constituencies such as the elderly organize to politicize health issues.

Reasons for rejecting The Himler Report.

One of the most salient points about the report is that, despite its apparent economic rationality, it has not been adopted by the AMA. The reason may precisely be its lack of political rationality. For one thing, its implementation may not be possible to achieve. Because of competition between the AMA and state medical societies for domination of practitioners, physicians might not submit to the discipline

[63] Max Weber, *Economy and Society: An Outline of Interpretive Sociology*, eds. Guenther Roth and Claus Wittich, 3 vols. (New York: Bedminster Press, 1968), pp. 1390-1392.

[64] Bertram Gross, "Friendly Fascism," *Social Policy* 1 (November-December 1971), p. 51.

of national organized medicine; and the AMA would not be able to deliver services to fulfill contractual agreements with the government. Second, there is apparently considerable question as to whether the AMA could retain control in policy making, should the government assume payment. The reformers evidently believe that the dictum "he who pays the piper calls the tune" is not necessarily true; the AMA leadership remains skeptical about the possibilities of professional domination of the government. In short, despite the reformers' insight into the potential increased income of government subsidies, increased income remains only a potential which may not be realizable. Third, governmental subsidies may not be as inevitable as the reformers believe. There is, as discussed above, the questionable political rationality of a redistribution of medical services in contemporary American society; and one can only note that, since Medicare and Medicaid, little further financial involvement of the federal government in the organization of medical services has taken place. To be sure, service redistribution plans have potential electoral value, but again, what is potential may not be politically realizable, for the support of the American public is uncertain. If, as in the case of Medicare, such plans are financed predominantly by the lower and middle classes through social security, these groups may well oppose such plans to prevent loss of real income— even though they are the very groups which most need such plans in time of illness. If financed through federal taxation, these plans may be opposed by these same groups if they believe that property and other taxes may be increased even further. In short, medical service redistribution plans may not be politically popular in view of the present class structure of payment for welfare services in American society.

Recapitulation

This chapter has examined a reform program proposed at the 1970 AMA national convention and found that, despite its manifest departure from the AMA's traditional monopolization strategy, the program is not only monopolistic but perhaps even more monopolistic than the old strategy. It proposes to organize physicians into more diversified and complex arrangements in order to gain increased income through new governmental subsidies. Nonetheless, tapping this new source of income requires increasing control over physicians, other health professionals, service-related administrative bodies, and various governmental institutions. Both increased income and control, however, are problematic because of a number of unfavorable political conditions: already successful physicians resistant to organized forms of practice, ruling groups politically uninterested in redistributing medical services among social classes, and the absence of an organized, widely-based popular constituency. While these unfavorable conditions may or may not change in the future, one must rest with the observation that, for now, the AMA has considered reform of the organization of the practice of medicine and has tentatively rejected it.

Conclusion

From a concern with the nature and the origins of contemporary institutions comes the question of why the practice of medicine has been institutionalized as a profession. Conventional sociological opinion on the matter has not been very illuminating. The classical essay on the medical profession by the American sociologist Talcott Parsons is inadequate, particularly because of its virtually nonexistent historical grounding and because of its unnecessary and unsupported assertions about the relationship between the medical profession's claims and the profession's actual activities. Parsons, for instance, underestimates the difficulty and complexity of providing technically efficacious medicine when he attempts to explain the profession's normative structure in terms of its capacity to optimize the delivery of good care. Moreover, he fails to consider the existence of controversy over the issue of how to organize medical care, apparently because he concentrates only on those norms of medical practice which correspond with his philosophy of what the norms of the profession should be.

Because medical care is very important to Parsons, so important, in fact, that he believes that medical care is necessary for the very functioning of the social system, he is too ready to assume that medicine's potential utility in maintaining the capacity of men to perform social roles could be the driving force behind the creation of the medical profession and of the structure of the profession's norms. Conspicuously absent in his thought are any sense of mechanism to link the alleged social role of the profession to its creation and any consideration that alternative forces might be responsible for the profession's institutionalization. Particularly lacking is any discussion of the role of physicians' interests in the institutionalization of the profession.

As an alternative approach to the problem, Max Weber's more comprehensive theory of economic and social action, as laid forth in *Economy and Society,* stands as an analysis of the role of monopolization and expansion in the institutionalization of *any* group. In many respects, monopolization is an applicable concept for the problem of the institutionalization of the medical profession, and it is possible to deduce what the organized conduct of the profession might be if it followed a tendency toward monopolization.

A review of substantive materials relevant to the problem of institutionalization initially turned to medical ethics, because they seemed to be the profession's answer to the problem of why men are conduced to pursue interests collectively rather than individually: fundamentally, it is made a matter of honor to do so. This idea had merit, since most if not virtually all modern medical ethics carried monopolistic consequences, even though presented in seemingly nonmonopolistic contexts. Medical ethics, however, have played other organizational roles as well. Some systems of medical ethics prior to the nineteenth century did not seem to lend themselves well to the creation of a monopolistic group, and some systems seemed to be concerned only with parochial professional organizations, rather than with members of the profession at large Some medical ethics played a political role as well; indeed, the political and organizational roles of medical ethics can even conflict at times. Many recent codes of the American Medical Association, for instance, seem to be caught in the dilemma of pushing for monopolization and yet trying to convince external observers that the profession is not monopolistic. In view of this finding, the question arises of why the profession has tended to present itself in a nonmonopolistic light, and exactly what the profession's external political requirements for monopolization have been. If the profession were not free to monopolize at will, what constraints had it encountered, and what mechanisms had been found to overcome them?

While it was possible at one point to speculate on which audiences the profession may have been addressing when it drew up revised codes of medical ethics, it became evident that a better appreciation of the political setting of the medical profession's institutionalization would require an in-depth historical analysis. Though I earlier treated the problem of the institutionalization of the profession more or less as for any group, I subsequently began a search for the origins and development of historically specific social phenomena: the medical organizations of England and the United States. I was most interested in finding out which historical concatenations provided the necessary conditions for the rise of the medical profession.

The rise of the medical profession did not occur in either nation until certain traditional political relationships passed away. In England, the Royal College of Physicians did not arise until the weakening of the traditional system of urban guilds and until the rise of an emergent state power, the monarch, willing to allow physicians to advance their collective interests despite traditions. In America, the medical profession never got very far with monopolizing activities until after the Revolution had assured political separation from England. In both, although in different forms, monopolistic organizations could not arise until new political forces were able to break the hold of traditional institutions.

The bestowal of monopolistic privileges to medical organizations, however, did not result in monopolization as a matter of course. On the contrary, these legally privileged groups were poor monopolizers and had, in time, to come to grips with the problems of persistent competition. This task was furthermore complicated by the rise of powerful anti-monopolistic ideologies. The result was the growth of new types of professional organization.

The first major model of authority for professional organization in Anglo-Saxon medicine was the Royal College of Physicians. The idea behind it was for a central organization manned by practitioners to rule over the great mass of practitioners, to direct their practice, to regulate entry into the profession, to seek out infringers on professional privileges, and to exact punishment. All legitimate practitioners were to be subject to an autonomous, self-regulating, self-policing, powerful disciplinary body. It was to be the ultimate arbiter in all matters relating to professional practice. Essentially, it was an attempt to transfer the concept of the guild to the profession, with the added proviso that all practitioners within the nation would be subject to its jurisdiction.

The RCP model was not stable. It was applied in both England and the early United States for a period of time, but in both cases, the RCP model did not prove adequate for the task. In England, it was replaced by the tripartite expanded model of the profession (physicians, surgeons, and apothecaries), and subsequently modified into a limited monopolistic form. In the United States, it was replaced in time by a decentralized confederation of local medical societies. The centralized English system placed control over the legal right to practice into the hands of the national government, while the American system handed control over entry into the profession to the state governments—nominally, it would appear. Insecure over lack of technical knowledge about medicine, governments typically left the administration of regulatory agencies, such as the General Medical Council and the state medical examination and licensing boards, to representatives of the official profession. As had frequently happened with other regulatory agencies,[1] the medical profession has apparently gained control over the agency intended to regulate it, indeed, legal authority over it.

In both the American and English cases, state involvement in the profession's institutions represented a solution to the failure of the profession to eliminate competitors adequately. The Royal College of Physicians had not converted its royal monopolistic privileges into an actual monopolization of the medical market, and the English courts gradually began to recognize the right of unlicensed practitioners to practice medicine. The courts did so, in part, because ineffective enforcement by the RCP allowed the rise of unlicensed but otherwise apparently competent practitioners. Justifying the RCP's monopolistic privileges became progressively more difficult, and finally the RCP willingly surrendered certain monopolistic privileges in exchange for sustained high pres-

---

[1] Henry W. Ehrmann, "Interest Groups and the Bureaucracy in Western Democracies," in Reinhard Bendix et al., eds., *State and Society: A Reader in Comparative Political Sociology* (Boston: Little, Brown, 1968), pp. 265-267.

tige. The result was the legalization of an already existing situation: a body of competent practitioners beyond the RCP's direct control. Henceforth, the profession was defined by the state's institutional representative, the GMC, and the profession's membership could be counted in the *Medical Register,* not on the RCP's roster.

In America, the fragmented system of political states resulted in a variegated professional structure. In general, however, those states with the most restrictive professional policies retained the right of entry in state administrative hands, while those with the least restrictive laws permitted medical societies to license physicians. Beset by antimonopolistic feeling and political turmoil, the medical societies gradually died out in the first half-century following the American Revolution. One major reason for their demise appears to have been, as in England, a failure to monopolize adequately. While official rhetoric denounced the fraudulent practitioner, a greater problem for the medical societies was posed by the medical-college-educated doctor, who took a diploma instead of a license. As medical colleges increased in number, the medical societies were unable to restrict entry into the profession, and restriction of membership became an impossibility. The separation of licensing from the medical societies by the state was eventually accomplished, and public fear of the subversion of medical affairs by the private control of the medical societies was allayed.

The creation of state medical institutions, then, could do what simple legal bestowal of monopolistic privilege could not. It helped answer charges that the private control of medicine would be used against the public interest, by arguing that the government would serve a watchdog function over the profession's actions. It increased the profession's prestige by adding political validation of the profession's claims of exclusive appropriation of correct knowledge. It provided licensed practitioners with a competitive advantage in the market, first by increasing the marginal utility of medical services through government approval, and second, in England, by providing inexpensive or free care at the point of delivery from those physicians eligible for state employment. And it explicitly made enforcement of restrictive measures a function of the government, not of the professional bodies. While policies might originate from the organized profession, administration could be carried out by governmental agencies and paid for by public funds. Unlike the profession, the state had the resources and administrative mechanisms for shaping the medical market in a monopolistic direction.

Both the inception of the profession and the conversion of monopolistic legal privileges into market advantages and controls were inextricably linked to the rise of state power. The greatest material advances of the profession were due to the profession-state liaison and not to "free enterprise" as understood in its laissez faire form. This state of affairs is understandable, since whatever weaknesses the nascent profession had in the marketplace could best be remedied by readily available state power. Even now, some reformers in the American Medical Association have shown interest in the advantages of state financing of medical care because of its potential superiority over the open market for making resources available, and its potential utility as a means for centralizing control over practitioners in the United States.

The question remains of why state power befriended the medical profession. While there may have been some general belief that the monopolistic devices which have been discussed, such as licensing, long medical curricula, and so forth, were merely instrumental mechanisms for upgrading the quality of medical practice, one cannot overlook the absence of institutional mechanisms for ensuring the distribution of medical care to those for whom it was technically indicated. The mechanisms for upgrading quality, as implemented, resulted in restriction of membership in the profession and increased inaccessibility to legitimate medical practitioners for certain social groups. Particularly in the United States, the development of the medical profession has been closely tied with the development of stratified relationships between social groups, so that quality medical care has tended to be a prized scarcity and an object of class behavior. Thus, explanations for the favorable treatment of the profession by the state are not entirely satisfactory when based on vague considerations such as the general social utility of more efficacious medical care, for they omit the role of the competition of social groups in larger society.

Essentially, I believe that the concept of a compatible constellation of interests between the medical profession as an organized institution and powerful social groups best explains the profession's successful institutionalization. To the degree that there is a favorable constellation of interests between the profession and elite groups, the collective interests of the profession can be furthered through progressive monopolization. It is for these reasons that I emphasize the explanatory role of the function of medical services for particular social groups rather than for society at large when considering the problem of professional institutionalization.

In this study I have been concerned with the problem of the factors which convert group monopolistic intent into successful monopolization. I have found five major types of considerations to be analytically useful: (1) the capacity of a group to order membership conduct in a monopolistic direction, (2) the capacity for a group to control membership size in a restrictionist direction, (3) the capacity for a group to eliminate competitive groups, (4) the favorability of a group's legal context, and (5) the favorability of a group's constellation of interests with powerful groups. Of these five, I am most impressed by the potential usefulness of the concept of the role of constellations of interests for research into problems of group success. Indeed, much of Weber's sociological theory of organization and domination is built on the perspective of the constellation of interests between interacting groups, with the concept of legitimacy perhaps taking a secondary role in certain respects.

Weber realized that social institutions are rarely if ever the product of any single group's interests but are usually the product of interaction among multiple social groups pursuing their interests. Institutions, then, persist because of the compromises of interest which powerful groups arrive at and seek to maintain on a tenuous basis. For Weber, constellations of interests explain why men with potentially competitive or conflicting interests engage in cooperative behavior. Weber also realized that men prefer to legitimize their privileges and benefits and so give to institutions a justification for existence absent in a mere constellation of interests. Legitimized institutional arrangements, in fact, take on the capacity to persist on a short-term basis, even when basic constellations of interests no longer support these arrangements. Phenomena such as authority are compensatory, short-term mechanisms for maintaining institutional relationships in the absence of favorable constellations of interests. Yet Weber, it would seem, would agree that institutional arrangements cannot long endure in the face of unstable or unfavorable constellations of interests. Even though claims of authority may smooth out and direct institutional functioning, constellations of interests are what most strongly commit men to institutional patterns.

I wish to decline at this time to make specific policy recommendations with respect to the organization of the medical profession or of health care delivery systems in either Britain or the United States. I simply have not conducted studies which provide the sort of information necessary to come to such conclusions. My study has been an analysis of how the medical profession has apparently been institutionalized and of the factors which influenced its institutionalization. Whether it should have been institutionalized in the form it has assumed or been institutionalized at all has not been my question. I have only wished to discriminate the types of monopolization patterns that the medical profession has followed and to investigate some of the conditions which led to the adoption of specific monopolization patterns. Indeed, in examining the problem of institutionalization, one becomes increasingly aware that the crucial issue is not whether a group pursues monopolization but the type of monopolization pattern it follows and the extent to which it is a successful monopolizer.

I hope, therefore, that any future studies of the medical profession, and policy studies in particular, take into account some recognition of the type of monopolization pattern which is contained in every organizational pattern. Studies which investigate the posibilities of the bureaucratization of practitioners — and these are very likely to appear, even if the term "bureaucratization" is not made explicit — should also take into account the monopolistic aspects of bureaucracy, for professionalization and bureaucratization are ultimately little more than alternative types of monopolization.

In the design of new systems for health care delivery, the role of the interests of practitioners should not be ignored, for it is one of the more important determinants of the type of monopolization pattern which is likely to be followed. Yet it is not the sole determinant. Even if the interests of patients, or of health care consumers, are not made felt on the system except as filtered through the interpretations of physicians, the interests of other groups than either patients or physicians may play an important role. While many alternative plausible systems of health care delivery can be designed with an eye to gratifying the interests of both patient and physician, they may not be politically realistic if the interests of ruling groups in society are not taken into account as well. The creation of a health care system is not simply an organizational problem; it is a political problem. Whatever the organizational "requirements" of such systems might be, they must find political acceptability if they are to be institutionalized. The social and political role of any health care delivery system may well be the most important determinant of the type of health institutions which will appear. One should not underestimate it.

Bibliography

Books

Anderson, Odin W. *The Uneasy Equilibrium*. New Haven, Conn.: College & University Press, 1968.

Andrews, Charles M. *The Colonial Period of American History*. Vol. I. New Haven and London: Yale University Press, 1934.

Aptheker, Herbert. *The Colonial Era*. New York: International Publishers, 1959.

Baldwin, William Lee. *Antitrust and the Changing Corporation*. Durham, N.C.: Duke University Press, 1961.

Bell, Whitfield J., Jr. *John Morgan: Continental Doctor*. Philadelphia: University of Pennsylvania Press, 1965.

Bendix, Reinhard. *Work and Authority in Industry*. New York and Evanston: Harper & Row, Publishers, 1956.

Bensman, Joseph. *Dollars and Sense*. New York: The Macmillan Company, 1967.

Benton, J.H., Jr.; Emerson, C.W.; and Buchanan, J.R. *Medical Freedom*. Boston, Mass.: The Massachusets Medical Liberty League, 1885.

Billroth, Theodor. *The Medical Sciences in the German Universities*. New York: The Macmillan Company, 1924.

Blanton, Wyndham B. *Medicine in Virginia in the Eighteenth Century*. Richmond: Garrett & Massie, Incorporated, 1931.

Boorstin, Daniel J. *The Americans: The Colonial Experience*. New York: Random House, 1958.

Brain, Lord Walter Russell. *Medicine and Government*. London: Tavistock Publications, 1967.

Bullough, Vern L. *The Development of Medicine as a Profession*. New York: Hafner Publishing Company, Inc., 1966.

Burn, W.L. *The Age of Equipoise*. New York: W.W. Norton & Company, Inc., 1964.

Burrage, Walter Lincoln. *A History of the Massachusetts Medical Society, 1781-1922*. Privately printed, 1923.

Burrow, James G. *A.M.A.: Voice of American Medicine*. Johns Hopkins Press, 1963.

Carr, A.S. Comyns; Garnett, W.H. Stuart; and Taylor, J.H. *National Insurance*. London: Macmillan and Co. Limited, 1912.

Carr-Saunders, A.M., and Wilson, P.A. *The Professions*. Oxford: The Clarendon Press, 1933.

Clark, Sir George. *A History of the Royal College of Physicians of London*. Oxford: Clarendon Press for the Royal College of Physicians. Two vols. 1964, 1966.

Clarke, Edward H., et al. *A Century of American Medicine: 1776-1876*. Brinklow, Maryland: Old Hickory Bookshop, 1962 (original edition 1876).

Clegg, H.A., and Chester, T.E. *Wage Policy and the Health Service*. Oxford: Basil Blackwell, 1957.

Cope, Zachary, ed. *Sidelights on the History of Medicine.* London: Butterworth and Co. (Publishers) Ltd., 1957.

Corner, George W. *Two Centuries of Medicine.* Philadelphia and Montreal: J.B. Lippincott Company, 1965.

Cowen, David L. *Medicine and Health in New Jersey: A History.* Princeton, N.J.: D. Van Nostrand Company, Inc., 1964.

Davis, Joseph Stancliffe. *Essays in the Earlier History of American Corporations: Eighteenth Century Business Corporations in the United States.* Two vols. New York: Russell & Russell, Inc., 1965.

Davis, N.S. *History of the American Medical Association from its Organization up to January, 1855.* Philadelphia: Lippincott, Grambo and Co., 1855.

———. *History of Medical Education and Institutions in the United States, From the First Settlement of the British Colonies to the Year 1850.* Chicago: S.C. Griggs & Co., Publishers, 1851.

Derbyshire, Robert C. *Medical Licensure and Discipline in the United States.* Baltimore and London: The Johns Hopkins Press, 1969.

Dubois, René. *Mirage of Health.* Garden City, New York: Anchor Books, Doubleday & Company, Inc., 1961.

Duffy, John, ed. *History of Medicine in Louisiana.* Two vols. Louisiana State University Press, 1962.

Eckstein, Harry. *The English Health Service: Its Origins, Structure, and Achievements.* Cambridge, Mass.: Harvard University Press, 1958.

Entralgo, Lain. *Doctor and Patient.* Translated from the Spanish by Frances Partridge. London: World University Library, Weidenfeld and Nicholson Ltd., 1969.

Erickson, Arvel B. *The Public Career of Sir James Graham.* Oxford: Basil Blackwell; Cleveland: The Press of Western Reserve University, 1952.

Feinbaum, Robert. "The Doctor and the Public: A Case Study of Professional Politics." Unpublished doctoral dissertation, Department of Sociology, University of California, Berkeley, 1967.

Fitz, Reginald H. *The Rise and Fall of the Licensed Physician in Massachusetts, 1781-1860.* Reprinted from Transactions of the Association of American Physicians, 1894.

Flint, Austin. *Medical Ethics and Etiquette.* New York: D. Appleton and Company, 1883.

Freidson, Eliot. *Profession of Medicine: A Study of the Sociology of Applied Knowledge.* New York: Dodd, Mead, 1970.

———. *Professional Dominance: the Social Structure of Medical Care.* New York: Atherton Press, 1970.

Friedman, Milton. *Capitalism and Freedom.* Chicago: University of Chicago Press, 1962.

Galdston, Iago. *Medicine in Transition.* Chicago and London: The University of Chicago Press, 1965.

Garceau, Oliver. *The Political Life of the American Medical Association.* Hamden, Conn.: Archon Books, 1961 (1941).

Gregory, John. *Lectures on the Duties and Qualifications of a Physician.* London: Strahan and T. Cadell, 1772.

Gruber, Georg B. *Arzt und Ethik.* Berlin: Walter de Gruyter & Co., 1948.
Guenzel, Louis. *Medical Ethics and Their Effect Upon the Public.* Privately published, 1950.
Harding, T. Swann. *The Degradation of Science.* New York: Farrar & Rinehart, Incorporated, 1931.
Hardwicke, H.J. *Medical Education and Practice.* Publisher unknown. 1880.
Harris, Richard. *A Sacred Trust.* New York: The New American Library, 1966.
Hofstadter, Richard. *Social Darwinism in American Thought.* Rev. Ed. Boston: Beacon Press, 1955.
Holmes, Oliver Wendell. *Medical Essays, 1842-1882.* Boston & New York: Houghton, Mifflin and Company, 1889.
Hooker, Worthington. *Dissertation on the Respect Due to the Medical Profession and the Reasons that It is Not Awarded By the Community.* Norwich, Conn.: J.G. Pooley, 1844.
———. *Physician and Patient: or, A Practical View of the Mutual Duties, Relations and Interests of the Medical Profession and the Community.* New York: Baker and Scribner, 1849.
Jenkins, Daniel T., ed. *The Doctor's Profession.* London: SCM Press Ltd., 1949.
Kaufman, Martin. *Homeopathy in America: The Rise and Fall of a Medical Heresy.* Baltimore and London: The Johns Hopkins Press, 1971.
Kett, Joseph F. *The Formation of the American Medical Profession: The Role of Institutions, 1780-1860.* New Haven and London: Yale University Press, 1968.
Konold, Donald E. *A History of American Medical Ethics 1847-1912.* Madison: University of Wisconsin Press, 1962.
Leake, Chauncey D., ed. *Percival's Medical Ethics.* Baltimore: Williams & Wilkins, 1927.
Letwin, William. *Law and Economic Policy in America: The Evolution of the Sherman Antitrust Act.* New York: Random House, 1965.
Levy, Hermann. *National Health Insurance.* Cambridge: At the University Press, 1944.
Lindsey, Almont. *Socialized Medicine in England and Wales: The N.H.S., 1948-1961.* Chapel Hill: University of North Carolina Press, 1962.
Little, Ernest Muirhead. *History of the British Medical Association 1832-1932.* London: British Medical Association, No date.
Lubove, Roy. *The Struggle for Social Security 1900-1935.* Cambridge, Mass.: Harvard University Press, 1968.
Lynch, Matthew, and Raphael, Stanley S. *Medicine and the State.* Springield, Ill.: Charles C. Thomas, 1963.
McCleary, G.F. *National Health Insurance.* London: H.K. Lewis & Co. Ltd., 1932.
Machlup, Fritz. *The Political Economy of Monopoly: Business, Labor, and Government Policies.* Baltimore: Johns Hopkins Press, 1952.
Marshall, T.H. *Class, Citizenship and Social Development.* Garden City,

New York: Anchor Books, Doubleday & Company, 1965.

Mathews, Joseph McDowell. *How to Succeed in the Practice of Medicine.* Louisville: Morton, 1902.

Millis, John S. *A Rational Public Policy for Medical Education and Its Financing.* New York: The National Fund for Radical Education, 1971.

Neale, A.D. *The Antitrust Laws of the United States of America: A Study of Competition Enforced by Law.* Cambridge: At the University Press, 1962.

Newman, Charles. *The Evolution of Medical Education in the Nineteenth Century.* London: Oxford University Press, 1957.

Palyi, Melchior. *Compulsory Medical Care and the Welfare State.* Chicago: The Heritage Foundation, Inc., 1949.

Parsons, Talcott. *The Social System.* London: The Free Press of Glencoe, 1951.

Platt, Sir Robert. *Doctor and Patient, Ethics, Morale, Government.* London: Nuffield Provincial Hospitals Trust, 1963.

Post, Alfred C.; Ely, William S.; Vanderpoel, S. Oakley; Pilcher, Lewis S.; Hunt, Thomas; Wey, William C.; Ordronaux, John; Roosa, Daniel B. St. John; Agnew, Cornelius R.; Jacobi, Abraham; and Hopkins, H.R. *An Ethical Symposium.* New York: G.P. Putnam's Sons, 1883.

Powell, J. Enoch. *A New Look at Medicine and Politics.* London: Pitman Medical Publishing Co. Ltd. 1966.

Poynter, F.N.L. *The Evolution of Medical Practice in Britain.* London: Pitman Medical Publishing Co. Ltd., 1961.

Rae, John. *Life of Adam Smith.* New York: Augustus M. Kelley, Bookseller, 1965 (1895).

Rayack, Elton. *Professional Power and American Medicine: The Economics of the American Medical Association.* Cleveland and New York: The World Publishing Company, 1967.

Reilley, Thomas F. *Building a Profitable Practice.* Philadelphia and London: J.B. Lippincott Company, 1912.

Richmond, Julius B. *Currents in American Medicine.* Cambridge Massachusetts: Harvard University Press, 1969.

Rivington, Walter. *The Medical Profession.* Dublin: Fannin & Co., 1879. 1879.

Ross, James Stirling. *The National Health Service in Great Britain: An Historical and Descriptive Study.* London, New York, Toronto: Oxford University Press, 1952.

Rozwenc, Edwin C., ed. *The Meaning of Jacksonian Democracy.* Boston: D.C. Heath and Company, 1963.

Schlesinger, Arthur M., Jr. *The Age of Jackson.* Boston: Little, Brown and Company, 1945.

Shafer, Henry Burnell. *The American Medical Profession, 1783-1850.* New York: AMS Press, 1936.

Shryock, Richard Harrison. *Medical Licensing in America, 1650-1965.* Baltimore, Maryland: The Johns Hopkins Press, 1967.

Somers, Anne R. *Hospital Regulation: The Dilemma of Public Policy.* Princeton, New Jersey: Princeton University Press, 1969.

Somers, Herman Miles, and Somers, Anne Ramsay. *Doctors, Patients, and Health Insurance: The Organization and Financing of Medical Care.* Washington, D.C.: The Brookings Institution, 1961.

Spivak, John L. *The Medical Trust Unmasked.* New York: Louis S. Siegfried, 1929.

Stevens, Rosemary. *American Medicine and the Public Interest.* New Haven: Yale University Press, 1971.

————. *Medical Practice in Modern England: The Impact of Specialization and State Medicine.* New Haven and London: Yale University Press, 1966.

Titmuss, Richard M. *Essays on "the welfare state".* New Haven: Yale University Press, 1959.

————. *Commitment to Welfare.* New York: Pantheon Books, 1968.

Vollmer, Howard M., and Mills, Donald L., eds. *Professionalization.* Englewood Cliffs, New Jersey: Prentice-Hall, Inc., 1966.

Walsh, James J. *History of Medicine in New York: Three Centuries of Medical Progress.* New York: National Americana Society, Inc., Vol. I., 1919.

Warner, Robert Stephen. "The Methodology of Max Weber's Comparative Studies." Unpublished doctoral dissertation, Department of Sociology, University of California, Berkeley, June, 1972.

Weber, Max. *Economy and Society: An Outline of Interpretive Sociology.* Edited by Guenther Roth and Claus Wittich. 3 vols. New York: Bedminster Press, 1968.

Wickes, Stephen. *History of Medicine in New Jersey, and of its Medical Men, From the Settlement of the Province to A.D. 1800.* Newark, N.J.: Martin R. Dennis & Co., 1879.

Wiebe, Robert H. *The Search for Order: 1877-1920.* New York: Hill and Wang,1967.

Willcocks, Arthur J. *The Creation of the N.H.S.: A Study of Pressure Group and a Major Social Policy Decision.* London: Routledge and Kegan Paul, 1967.

Ziemssen, Oswald. *Die Ethik des Arztes.* Leipzig: Verlag von Georg Thieme, 1899.

Articles

Ackerknecht, E.H. "Zur Geschichte der medizinischen Ethik." *Praxis* 17 (1964), pp. 578-581.

Bronson, Henry. "Historical Account of the Origin of the Connecticut Medical Society." *Proceedings of Connecticut Medical Society*, May 1973, pp. 53-62.

Cheever, David W. "Medicine as a Profession." *Boston Medical and Surgical Journal*, 135 (24 December 1896), pp. 637-641.

Cowen, David L. "Liberty, Laissez-Faire and Licensure in Nineteenth Century Britain." *Bulletin of the History of Medicine*, 43 (January-February 1969), pp. 30-40.

Cutler, Lloyd N., and staff. "The Legislative Monopolies Achieved by Small Businesses." *Yale Law Journal*, 48 (March 1939), pp. 847-858.

Edelstein, Ludwig. "The Hippocratic Oath." *Bulletin of the History of Medicine*, Supplement 1 (1943), pp. 1-64.

Ehrmann, Henry W. "Interest Groups and the Bureaucracy in Western

Democracies," in Reinhard Bendix et al., eds., *State and Society: A Reader in Comparative Political Sociology*. Boston: Little, Brown and Company, 1968.

Fisher, William R. "Legal Restriction of Medical Practice." *The Arena*, 19 (1898), pp. 527-534.

Fitts, William T., Jr., and Fitts, Barbara. "Ethical Standards of the Medical Profession." *The Annals of the American Academy of Political and Social Science*, 297 (January 1955), pp. 118-124.

Fitz, Reginald H. "The Legislative Control of Medical Practice." *Boston Medical and Surgical Journal*, 130 (June 1894), pp. 581-585, 609-613, 637-641. 131 (July 1894), pp. 1-5, 25-27.

Garceau, Oliver. "The Morals of Medicine." *The Annals of the American Academy of Political and Social Science*, 363 (January 1966), pp. 60-69.

Gross, Bertram. "Friendly Fascism." *Social Policy*, 1 (November-December 1971), pp. 44-52.

Hughes, Everett C. "The Professions in Society." *Canadian Journal of Economics and Political Science*, 26 (February 1960), pp. 54-61.

Huxley, T. H. "The State and the Medical Profession." *Nineteenth Century*, 15 (1884), pp. 228-230.

Hyde, David R., and staff. "The American Medical Association: Power, Purpose, and Politics in Organized Medicine." *Yale Law Journal*, 63 (May 1954), pp. 938-1022.

Kessel, Reuben A. "Price Discrimination in Medicine." *Journal of Law and Economics*, 1 (1958), pp. 20-53.

Lashley, Miriam, et al. "Group Health Plans: Some Legal and Economic Aspects." *Yale Law Journal*, 53 (1943), pp. 162-182.

Lister, John. "By the London Post." *New England Journal of Medicine*, 285 (25 November 1971), pp. 1247-1249.

MacIver, R. M. "The Social Significance of Professional Ethics." *The Annals of the American Academy of Political and Social Science*, 297 (January 1955), pp. 118-124.

Naylor, Mildred V. "A New Jersey Petition." *Bulletin of the History of Medicine*, 17 (1945), pp. 93-100.

Parsons, Talcott. "On the Concept of Political Power." *Proceedings of the American Philosophical Society*, 107 (June 1963), pp. 232-262.

———. "Social Change and Medical Organization in the United States: A Sociological Perspective." *The Annals of the American Academy of Political and Social Science*, 356 (March 1963), pp. 21-33.

———. "The Professions and Social Structure." In *Essays in Sociological Theory*, rev. ed., pp. 34-39. London: The Free Press of Glencoe, Collier-Macmillan Ltd., 1954.

Posner, Richard, et al. "Judicially Compelled Admission to Medical Societies: The Falcone Case." *Harvard Law Review*, 75 (1962), pp. 1186-1198.

Radbill, Samuel X. "A History of Medical Ethics." *Philadelphia Medicine*, 13 July 1962, pp. 873-876.

Rosen, George. "Fees and Fee Bills: Some Economic Aspects of Medical Practice in Nineteenth Century America." *Bulletin of the History of Medicine*, Supplement 6 (1946), pp. 1-91.

Simmel, Georg. "The Secret Society." In *The Sociology of Georg Simmel*, edited by Kurt H. Wolff, pp. 345-376. London: The Free Press of Glencoe, Collier-Macmillan Ltd., 1950.

Smithies, Frank. "On the Origin and Development of Ethics in Medicine and the Influence of Ethical Formulae upon Medical Practice." *Annals of Clinical Medicine*, 3 (March 1925), pp. 573-603.

Steiner, Walter Ralph. *the Evolution of Medicine in Connecticut, with the Foundation of the Yale Medical School as its Notable Achievement*. No publisher. 1914.

Womack, Nathan A. "The Evolution of the National Board of Medical Examiners." *J.A.M.A.*, 192 (June 1965), pp. 817-823.

Wood, Henry. "Medical Slavery Through Legislation." *The Arena*, 8 (1893), pp. 680-689.

Other sources

"Actions Taken by the AMA House of Delegates at Its Recent Annual Convention." American Medical Association. Mimeographed copy. 13 July 1970.

"Health Care: Rx for Change." *Saturday Review*, 53 (22 August 1970), entire issue.

"Principles of Medical Ethics." American Medical Association. VI-VII. 1957.

"Principles of Medical Ethics." *J.A.M.A.*, 140 (25 June 1949), pp. 700-703.

"Report of Coordinating Committee." *J.A.M.A.*, 140 (25 June 1949), pp. 694-699.

"Report of the Council on Planning and Development (The Himler Report)." American Medical Association. Mimeographed copy. July 1970.

Interview with Peter Libby, medical student delegate to annual American Medical Association convention in Chicago, Illinois, 1970; conducted on several occasions during August 1970.

Personal communication from Timothy B. Norbeck, assistant director, Department of Specialty Society Services, American Medical Association, 7 June 1972.

Index

317